QBASE PAEDIATRICS 3
MCQS FOR THE PART B MRCPCH

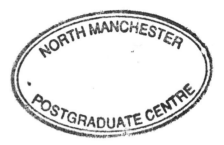

QBASE PAEDIATRICS 3
MCQS FOR THE PART B MRCPCH

Rachel U. Sidwell
MRCP, MRCPH, DFFP, DA

Mike Thomson
FRCP, FRCPH, DCH, MD

with contributions from James S. A. Green, FRCS, LLM,
Whipps Cross Hospital and Jamie Carter, BSc, MRCPCH,
DTM&H, Lambeth PCT

QBase developed and edited by
Edward Hammond

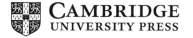
CAMBRIDGE
UNIVERSITY PRESS

CAMBRIDGE UNIVERSITY PRESS
Cambridge, New York, Melbourne, Madrid, Cape Town, Singapore, São Paulo, Delhi

Cambridge University Press
The Edinburgh Building, Cambridge CB2 8RU, UK

Published in the United States of America by Cambridge University Press, New York

www.cambridge.org
Information on this title: www.cambridge.org/9780521698375

© Cambridge University Press 2008

First published 2008

Printed in the United Kingdom at the University Press, Cambridge

A catalogue record for this publication is available from the British Library

Library of Congress Cataloguing in Publication Data

Sidwell, Rachel U.
QBase paediatrics 3: MCQs for the Part B MRCPCH / Rachel U. Sidwell, Mike Thomson;
with contributions from James S. A. Green and Jamie Carter; QBase developed
and edited by Edward Hammond.
p. ; cm.
Includes bibliographical references and index.
ISBN 978-0-521-69837-5 (pbk.)
1. Pediatrics–Examinations, questions, etc. I. Thomson, Mike (Mike Andrew)
II. Green, James S. A. III. Carter, Jamie. IV. Hammond, Edward. V. Title.
[DNLM: 1. Pediatrics–Examination Questions. WS 18.2 S569q 2008]
RJ48.2.S33 2008
618.9200076–dc22   2008006055

ISBN 978-0-521-69837-5 paperback

Contents

Preface

The questions in this book focus on areas of child health relevant to those training as paediatricians. This book is an aid for those taking the MRCPCH.

The questions in this book are multiple true-false questions (MCQs) which are also available on the accompanying CD Rom allowing practice in this component of the exam, which is the key to passing MCQs, and also makes it a little more fun. The CD Rom allows the questions to be randomly scrambled, and also for methodical learning, questions on a particular subject can be selected separately, and a single topic covered in detail. In addition there are a few example questions of 'best of five' and 'extended match' type questions included at the end of each 'exam' in the book.

The MRCPCH Part I exam consists of Paper One A and Paper One B. Paper One B forms part of the MRCPCH Part One examination. The exam format will be changing again (and it is advisable to check the college website www.rcpch.ac.uk/examinations, for any further changes). Since January 2008 both paper 1A and paper 1B will consist of 69 questions made up of the following;

25 Multiple true-false questions (MCQ)

35 Best of five questions (BOF)

9 Extended match questions (EMQ)

Remember to read each question carefully, and do not caught out by simple phraseology. Look out for key phrases such as 'always' and 'never' both of which are unlikely to be true. Terms such as 'commonly', 'usually' and 'often' are unfortunately ambiguous and open to interpretation. And finally remember that even if you think you know nothing about a question, you must answer as intelligently as you can because your probability of being right is more than that of being wrong, simply because you are making an educated guess.

Have fun, and best of luck!

Installation Instructions

QBASE PAEDIATRICS 3 ON CD-ROM MINIMUM SYSTEM REQUIREMENTS

- An IBM compatible PC with a 80386 processor and 4 MB of RAM
- VGA monitor set up to display at least 256 colours
- CD-ROM drive
- Windows 95 or higher with Microsoft compatible mouse

NB: The display setting of your computer must be set to display 'SMALL FONTS' (see MS Windows manuals for further instructions on how to do this if necessary)

INSTALLATION INSTRUCTIONS

The program will install the appropriate files onto your hard drive. It requires the QBase CD-ROM to be in installed in the CD-ROM drive (usually drives D: or E:).

In order to run QBase, the CD must be in the drive

Print **Readme.txt** and **Helpfile.txt** on the CD-ROM for fuller instructions and user manual

WINDOWS 95, 98, 2000, XP

1. Insert the QBase CD-ROM into the drive
2. From the Start Menu, select the Run ... option, type **D:\setup.exe** (where D: is the CD-ROM drive) and press OK or open the contents of the CD-ROM and double-click the **setup.exe** icon
3. Follow the 'Full – install all files' to accept the default directory for installation of QBase
4. Click 'Yes' to the prompt 'Do you want setup to create Program Manager groups?' If you have a previously installed version of QBase, click 'Yes' to the next prompt 'Should the new Program Manager groups replace existing duplicate groups?'
5. To run QBase, go to the Start Menu, then Programs, QBase and **QBase Exam**. From Windows Explorer, double-click the **QBase.exe** file in the QBase folder on your hard drive.

Note on QBase

Notes for users of *QBase Paediatrics 3* on CD-ROM

Please read carefully and print the HELPFILE on the QBase CD-ROM as it contains detailed information on the features and analysis functions of QBase.

QBase is an interactive MCQ examination program designed to help candidates improve their performance in MCQs. Please follow the installation instructions printed on the previous page. Once installed, the QBase program resides on your hard disk and reads the data from whatever QBase CD is in your CD drive. If you install QBase from this CD, it will update any previous version of the program. Owners of previous QBase titles will then have access to any new functions available on this new version of the program. All QBase CDs will work with the new program. To check for successful installation of the new program, check the Quick Start Menu screen: it should have 5 exam buttons.

QBase Paediatrics 3 contains 300 questions for the Part B MRCPH. The 'Autoset Exam' option on this CD will present you with an exam of 60 questions, utilizing any of the 300 questions on the CD. The 5 predefined exams on the CD are constructed in the same way, and are exactly the same as the 5 exams printed in this book. You can also generate your own customized exams using the 'Create your own exam' option. You can save completed exams and your responses to your hard disk, allowing you to review or resit the same paper at a later stage in your revision. Please refer to the helpfile on the CD for more information. To further enhance your revision, instead of selecting the 'Resit exam' option, we suggest that you try the 'Resit shuffled exam' option. The leaves within each question will then be randomly shuffled, removing your ability to remember the pattern of correct answers rather than the facts. The exam analysis functions of QBase will provide you with a detailed breakdown of your performance.

Abbreviations

ACTH	adrenocorticotrophic hormone
ADH	antidiuretic hormone
ALT	alanine aminotransferase
ANA	antinuclear antibody
APTT	activated partial thromboplastin time
ASD	atrial septal defect
AST	aspartate aminotransferase
AV node	atrioventricular node
BCG	Bacille Calmette-Guérin
CAM	cystic adenomatoid malformation
CHD	congenital heart disease
CMV	cytomegalovirus
CNS	central nervous system
CSF	cerebrospinal fluid
CT	computed tomography
DIC	disseminated intravascular dissemination
DNA	deoxyribonucleic acid
2,3 DPG	2,3-diphosphoglycerate
ECG	electrocardiogram
EEG	electro-encephalogram
FSH	follicle-stimulating hormone
GABA	gamma aminobutyric acid
GCSF	granulocyte-colony-stimulating factor
GNRH	gonadotrophin-releasing hormone
G6PD	glucose-6 phosphate dehydrogenase
Hb	haemoglobin
HCG	human chorionic gonadotrophin
HHV-6	human herpes virus 6
HIV	human immunodeficiency virus
IGF-1	insulin-like growth factor-1
IUGR	intrauterine growth retardation
JIA	juvenile idiopathic arthritis
LFTs	liver function tests
LGB	lateral geniculate body
LH	luteinizing hormone
MMR	Measles, mumps, rubella
MRI	magnetic resonance imaging

PCR	polymerase chain reaction
PTH	parathyroid hormone
SLE	systemic lupus erythematosus
TB	tuberculosis
TPN	total parenteral nutrition
TSH	thyroid-stimulating hormone
VSD	ventricular septal defect
VZIG	varicella zoster immunoglobulin

Q 1. **The following are true of X-linked recessive disorders**

   A. Females are unaffected

   B. Sons of affected males have a 100% chance of being affected

   C. Sons of female carriers have a 25% chance of being affected

   D. Daughters of affected males have a 100% chance of being carriers

   E. Daughters of female carriers have a 50% chance of being carriers

Q 2. **Recognized features of Marfan syndrome include**

   A. Lens subluxation, usually downwards

   B. Femoral hernia

   C. Learning disability

   D. Hemivertebrae

   E. Autosomal recessive inheritance

Q 3. **Apert syndrome is characterized by**

   A. Syndactyly

   B. Polydactyly

   C. Acne

   D. Irregular craniosynostosis

   E. Mental deficiency

Q 4. **In achondroplasia, the following problems may develop**

   A. Upper airway obstruction

   B. Cord compression

   C. Hydrocephalus

   D. Osteoarthritis

   E. Sensorineural deafness

Q 5. The following are true

    A. Somatic cells contain 23 pairs of autosomes
    B. Gametes are haploid
    C. The bases cytosine and adenine pair together
    D. Adenine is a pyrimidine nitrogenous base
    E. In DNA replication, new base pairs are added to the 5′ end of the single DNA strand

Q 6. Regarding the optic (second) cranial nerve

    A. It is derived embryologically from the hind-brain
    B. It has both an intra-orbital and intracranial component
    C. The fibres from the lateral half of the retina cross over at the optic chiasma to the optic tract of the opposite side
    D. The majority of the fibres in the optic tract end in the medial geniculate body
    E. The upper half of the retina is represented on the lower lip of the calcerian fissure of the visual cortex

Q 7. Parasympathetic nervous system stimulation causes

    A. Stimulation of the detrusor muscle of the bladder
    B. Pilo-erection
    C. Uterine contraction
    D. Bronchial constriction
    E. Activation of peristalsis

Q 8. Regarding neural tube defects

    A. There is an association with isotretinoin taken during pregnancy
    B. The recurrence risk after two previous infants with neural tube defects is 10%
    C. Reduced alpha-fetoprotein (α-FP) is present in the amniotic fluid
    D. Spina bifida occulta is not associated with neurological symptoms
    E. Neural tube closure takes place in the fourth week of intrauterine life

Q 9. Lennox-Gastaut syndrome

    A. Presents with malabsorption
    B. Is a cause of developmental regression

C. Responds well to vitamin supplementation
D. Has autosomal recessive inheritance
E. Is more common in Down's syndrome

Q 10. **The following are side-effects of phenytoin**

A. Hyperphagia
B. Peripheral retinal atrophy
C. Hirsutism
D. Acne
E. Rickets

Q 11. **Concerning juvenile myoclonic epilepsy**

A. The seizures are partial
B. A quarter of patients have a positive family history of epilepsy
C. The gene has been identified on chromosome 7
D. Phenytoin is the treatment of choice
E. Photic stimulation increases positive EEG findings by over 30%

Q 12. **A normal 5-year-old is able to**

A. Do all their buttons up
B. Hop
C. Tie shoelaces
D. Say their home address
E. Copy a cross

Q 13. **Iris coloboma is seen in**

A. Down's syndrome
B. Turner syndrome
C. Rubinstein-Taybi syndrome
D. Trisomy 13
E. Klinefelter's syndrome

Q 14. **The following are causes of a large pupil**

A. Holmes-Adie pupil
B. Congenital rubella syndrome
C. Lowe's oculocerebrorenal syndrome
D. Ecstacy
E. Fabry's disease

Q 15. The following are true of the oxyhaemoglobin dissociation curve

    A. At the p50 the surrounding partial pressure of oxygen is normally 27 mmHg
    B. In mixed venous blood the oxygen saturation is 50%
    C. Methaemoglobinaemia decreases the affinity of haemoglobin for oxygen
    D. Cyanotic congenital heart disease does not affect the curve
    E. Hypothermia increases the affinity of haemoglobin for oxygen

Q 16. The following may be seen in the blood film in iron deficiency anaemia

    A. Target cells
    B. Anisocytosis
    C. Pencil cells
    D. Thrombocytopenia
    E. Increased free erythrocyte porphyrin

Q 17. The following cause splenomegaly with resultant anaemia

    A. Niemann-Pick disease
    B. Langerhans cell histiocytosis
    C. Portal hypertension
    D. Thalassaemia major
    E. Immune haemolytic anaemia

Q 18. These hereditary disorders predispose a child to thrombosis

    A. Protein C deficiency
    B. Hermansky-Pudlak syndrome
    C. Antithrombin III deficiency
    D. Bernard-Soulier syndrome
    E. Factor V Leiden deficiency

Q 19. Concerning laboratory investigations of a bleeding disorder

    A. Von Willebrand's disease has a prolonged APTT
    B. Prothrombin time (PT) is prolonged in haemophilia B
    C. Bleeding time is prolonged in haemophilia A
    D. Prolonged bleeding time occurs with impaired platelet numbers

E. APTT is sensitive to factors in the intrinsic coagulation pathway

Q 20. **The following conditions are primary T-cell deficiencies**

    A. Adenosine deaminase deficiency
    B. Hereditary angioneurotic oedema
    C. Wiskott-Aldrich syndrome
    D. MHC class II deficiency
    E. Chronic granulomatous disease

Q 21. **In staphylococcal scalded skin syndrome**

    A. The child is generally well
    B. It is usually due to *Staphylococcus aureus* group I phages
    C. The skin loss is superficial
    D. It is most common in school age children
    E. Frozen section of skin may help the diagnosis

Q 22. **Regarding galactosaemia**

    A. It causes an inability to metabolize galactose
    B. It causes an inability to metabolize lactose
    C. It is X-linked recessive
    D. It causes dysarthria
    E. Ovarian failure is a feature

Q 23. **In Hartnup disease**

    A. It is usually asymptomatic in children
    B. It is a cause of ataxia
    C. There is a photosensitive rash
    D. The acylcarnitine profile of a blood spot is diagnostic
    E. There is an accumulation of tryptophan

Q 24. **Medium Chain Acyl CoA Dehydrogenase Deficiency (MCADD)**

    A. Is a urea cycle defect
    B. Affects up to 1 in 40 of the UK population as asymptomatic carriers
    C. May present with encephalopathy
    D. Causes hepatomegaly
    E. Shows a characteristic urine amino acid profile

Exam 1

Questions

Q 25. **In paediatric liver disease, portal hypertension**

    A. Occurs when portal pressure is elevated to 10–12 mmHg
    B. Results in cephalic flow of collaterals inferior to the umbilicus
    C. May cause signs of spinal compression
    D. May result from factor V Leiden deficiency
    E. Should be treated prophylactically with propranolol in children under the age of 4 years

Q 26. **Hirschsprung's disease**

    A. Is inherited in an autosomal recessive fashion
    B. Is due to unopposed parasympathetic activity in the affected segment of the bowel
    C. Has an equal incidence in girls and boys
    D. Is seen more frequently in children with Down's syndrome than in the general population
    E. Presents in more than 80% in the neonatal period

Q 27. **The following occur more commonly in Crohn's disease than ulcerative colitis**

    A. Erythema nodosum
    B. Pyoderma gangrenosum
    C. Ankylosing spondyloarthropathy with HLA B27
    D. Uveitis
    E. Cholangiocarcinoma

Q 28. **Recognized features of Alagille's syndrome include**

    A. Tuberous xanthomas and raised serum cholesterol
    B. Progression to cirrhosis and chronic liver failure requiring liver transplantation
    C. Aortic stenosis
    D. Tetralogy of Fallot
    E. Abnormalities of peroxisomal function

Q 29. **In chronic liver disease in childhood, the following are correct**

    A. Spironolactone is useful in the treatment of ascites at any age
    B. A low plasma cholesterol is an adverse prognostic feature
    C. Sleep reversal occurs as a feature of hepatic encephalopathy

    D. There is an increased overall incidence of Hirschsprungs's disease
    E. Spontaneous bacterial peritonitis is a potentially fatal complication of ascites

Q 30. In the fetal circulation

    A. Oxygenated blood is transported to the fetus via the umbilical artery
    B. The ductus venosus drains into the superior vena cava
    C. Oxygenated blood passes through the foramen ovale from the right to the left side of the heart
    D. There is no significant blood flow through the coronary arteries
    E. Blood flows from the pulmonary artery via the ductus arteriosus into the descending aorta

Q 31. Chromosome 22q11 microdeletion is associated with the following forms of congenital heart disease

    A. Truncus arteriosus
    B. Patent ductus arteriosus
    C. Dissecting aortic aneurysm
    D. Peripheral pulmonary stenosis
    E. Tetralogy of Fallot

Q 32. Torsades de Pointes may be caused by

    A. Organophosphate poisoning
    B. Aspirin
    C. Anorexia nervosa
    D. Hypomagnesaemia
    E. Lead poisoning

Q 33. The following features would be consistent with the murmur of a ventricular septal defect

    A. Wide fixed splitting of the second heart sound
    B. Loudest at the upper left sternal edge
    C. Mid-diastolic apical murmur
    D. Parasternal thrill
    E. Loud P2

Q 34. Congenital complete heart block

A. Always requires treatment with a pacemaker
B. Is associated with Turner syndrome
C. May be secondary to an atrioventricular septal defect
D. Is associated with maternal anti-Ro antibodies
E. May present with hydrops fetalis

Q 35. Causes of an acidosis with a normal anion gap are

A. Lactic acidosis
B. Ketoacidosis
C. Salicylate poisoning
D. Proximal renal tubular acidosis
E. Diarrhoea

Q 36. Causes of Fanconi's syndrome include

A. Hypoparathyroidism
B. Cystinosis
C. Glue-sniffing
D. Galactosaemia
E. Wilson's disease

Q 37. Haemolytic uraemic syndrome

A. Causes hypokalaemia
B. Involves a sideroblastic anaemia
C. May be caused by salmonella
D. If familial, has a better prognosis
E. Is the most common cause of renal failure in children in the UK

Q 38. The features of Alport syndrome are

A. Haematuria
B. Proptosis
C. Cataract
D. Asymmetrical craniosynostosis
E. Hyperphagia

Q 39. Regarding surfactant

A. It decreases lung compliance at low lung volumes
B. There is a lower incidence of pneumothorax with natural surfactant than synthetic surfactant

C. It decreases the need for oxygen in infants with respiratory distress syndrome

D. It can cause a transient decrease in oxygen saturation when given

E. It helps maintain the functional residual capacity of the lungs

Q 40. Cystic fibrosis

A. Causes a hyperkalaemic alkalosis

B. Is a cause of intussusception

C. Is due to a mutation in the cystic fibrosis transmembrane regulator (*CFTR*) gene on chromosome 8

D. Is a cause of nasal polyps

E. Is due to a defect in the sodium channels

Q 41. Oligoarticular Juvenile idiopathic arthritis

A. Has an equal sex ratio

B. Goes on to affect more than four joints after 6 months in 50% of cases

C. Is rheumatoid factor (RhF) positive

D. Typically affects the hands and feet

E. If associated with uveitis, may progress silently to blindness

Q 42. Inguinal hernias

A. Are usually direct in children

B. Are more common in females in childhood

C. Are associated with Marfan syndrome

D. Are more common on the right side

E. Are associated with prematurity

Q 43. Octreotide

A. Is a GNRH analogue

B. Is used in the treatment of insulinoma

C. Causes irreversible alopecia

D. Commonly causes altered liver function tests

E. Is effective as an anti-emetic in palliative care

Q 44. Mycophenolate mofetil

A. Is a calcineurin inhibitor

B. Can cause hypertension

C. Has a lower incidence of side-effects in children
D. Is an inactive precursor
E. May cause pancreatitis

Q 45. The side-effects of doxorubicin include

A. Mucositis (uncommonly)
B. Supraventricular tachycardia
C. Cardiomyopathy at low dosage
D. Pulmonary fibrosis
E. Retinopathy

Q 46. Physical features seen in anorexia nervosa include

A. Acidosis
B. Low growth hormone
C. Low rT3
D. Raised LH
E. Short QT interval on ECG

Q 47. Regarding multiple pregnancy

A. The incidence of monozygotic twins is 1 in 1000 pregnancies
B. There is a 1 in 33 spontaneous rate for dizygotic twins
C. There is an increased risk of congenital anomalies among monozygotic twins
D. Dizygotic twins always have a dichorionic placenta
E. Dichorionic twins are at risk of twin-twin transfusion syndrome

Q 48. Neonatal pulmonary haemorrhage is associated with

A. Pneumonia
B. Acute cardiac failure
C. Respiratory distress syndrome
D. Prematurity
E. Asphyxia

Q 49. In osteopenia of prematurity

A. Inadequate milk intake is a risk factor
B. Large for gestational age is a risk factor
C. Clinical rickets is commonly seen

D. Serum calcium is low

E. Serum PTH is high

Q 50. The following maternal factors are associated with increased neonatal serum bilirubin levels

A. Diabetes

B. Hypertension

C. Greek race

D. Black race

E. Smoking

Q 51. The following are true regarding neonatal nutrition

A. Preterm infants need approximately 180 kcal/kg/day

B. Infants with chronic lung disease have increased calorific requirements

C. Lactose is better absorbed than glucose polymers in preterm infants

D. Breast milk has a higher lactose content than cow's milk

E. Breast-feeding reduces the incidence of osteoporosis in the mother

Q 52. Clinical features of the syndrome of inappropriate antidiuretic hormone secretion (SIADH) include

A. Sacral oedema

B. Confusion

C. Hypertension

D. Personality change

E. Seizures

Q 53. The following are true of insulins

A. Ultra-short acting insulin has a peak action at 0.5 hours

B. Short-acting insulin has an onset of 0.5 hours

C. Short-acting insulin has a duration of 2–3 hours

D. Medium-acting insulin has a duration of 10–12 hours

E. Ultra-short acting insulin has an onset of 2 minutes

Q 54. Congenital hypothyroidism

A. Is usually of autosomal recessive inheritance

B. Is more common in males

Exam 1

Questions

C. Is a cause of neonatal abdominal distension

D. May be associated with normal intelligence

E. Is often associated with goitre

Q 55. **In congenital adrenal hyperplasia due to 21-hydroxylase deficiency the following are elevated**

A. Cortisol

B. Aldosterone

C. Testosterone

D. Androstenedione

E. ACTH

Q 56. **The following are true regarding congenital adrenal hyperplasia**

A. Boys are likely to be diagnosed earlier than girls

B. They are a group of autosomal dominant disorders due to defects in the biosynthesis of cortisol

C. More than 80% of cases are due to 11-hydroxylase deficiency

D. A late-onset form presents in pubertal girls with menstrual irregularity and hirsutism

E. 3-β-hydroxysteroid dehydrogenase deficiency causes hypertension

Q 57. **The following are live attenuated vaccines**

A. Pertussis

B. Influenza

C. Typhoid

D. Diphtheria

E. Yellow fever

Q 58. **Regarding *Giardia* infection**

A. Children with chronic pancreatitis are more susceptible to infection

B. Infection may be asymptomatic

C. It is a cause of chronic malabsorption

D. It may cause partial villous atrophy

E. It usually causes bloody diarrhoea

Q 59. Mumps infection

    A. Infectivity is from 1 week after the parotid swelling appears
    B. Usually results in unilateral parotitis
    C. Causes subclinical infection in 60% of cases
    D. Has an incubation period of 7–10 days
    E. Is most common in the autumn

Q 60. Roseola infantum

    A. Causes red papules on the uvula and soft palate
    B. Causes eyelid oedema
    C. May cause clinical confusion with measles infection
    D. Is a common cause of febrile convulsions in young children
    E. Usually has no prodrome

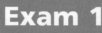

A 1.   **A.** false   **B.** false   **C.** false   **D.** true   **E.** true

Females can be affected as carriers due to random X inactivation (Lyonization). There is no father-to-son transmission. Sons of female carriers have a 50% chance of being affected.

A 2.   **A.** false   **B.** true   **C.** true   **D.** true   **E.** false

Marfan syndrome is due to a mutation within the fibrillin gene (*FBN1*) on chromosome 15, and is an autosomal dominant condition. Lens subluxation is usually upwards. Femoral hernia and hemivertebrae are occasionally seen. Learning disability is present in around 40% of cases.

A 3.   **A.** true   **B.** false   **C.** true   **D.** true   **E.** true

Apert syndrome is an irregular craniosynostosis due to mutations in the fibroblast growth factor receptor 2 gene (*FGFR2*) on chromosome 10. The major other features are mental deficiency, short stature, typical facies (hypertelorism, shallow orbits, downslanting palpebral fissures, full forehead) and syndactyly.

A 4.   **A.** true   **B.** true   **C.** true   **D.** false   **E.** false

Upper airways obstruction can occur due to the craniofacial abnormalities. Cord compression, though rare, can happen as a consequence of spinal canal stenosis, kyphosis and disc lesions, and a small foramen magnum. Due to the short Eustachian tubes, conductive hearing loss secondary to recurrent middle ear infection may be seen.

A 5.   **A.** false   **B.** true   **C.** false   **D.** false   **E.** false

Somatic cells contain 22 pairs of autosomes and 1 pair of sex chromosomes, and are diploid. The gametes are haploid and therefore contain half the number of chromosomes (22 autosomes and 1 sex chromosome). Cytosine pairs with guanine. Cytosine and thymidine are pyrimidines, and adenine and guanine are purines. New base pairs are added to the 3′ end of the DNA strand.

A 6.   **A.** false   **B.** true   **C.** false   **D.** false   **E.** false

The optic nerve is derived embryologically from the fore-brain. At the optic chiasma the fibres from the lateral half of the retina (nasal visual field) pass back in the optic tract of the same side, while the fibres from the medial half of the retina (temporal visual field) cross over to the optic tract of the opposite side. The majority of the fibres of the optic tract end in the lateral geniculate body of the thalamus. The occipital visual cortex is located above and below the calcerian fissure. The upper and lower halves of the retina are represented on the upper and lower lips of the calcerian fissure respectively.

Anatomy for Anaesthetists. Ed. Ellis H & Feldman S, 6th edn 1993, Oxford: Blackwell Science, pp. 253–6.

A 7.   **A.** true   **B.** false   **C.** false   **D.** true   **E.** true

The actions of the parasympathetic nervous system are those of the body when not under stress. Stimulation of the parasympathetic nervous system causes stimulation of the bladder detrusor muscle, uterine vasodilatation, bronchial constriction and activation of peristalsis. Stimulation of the sympathetic nervous system causes pilo-erection, uterine contraction and vasoconstriction, bronchial dilatation and inhibition of peristalsis.

Anatomy for Anaesthetists. Ed. Ellis H & Feldman S, 6th edn 1993, Oxford: Blackwell Science p. 231.

A 8.   **A.** false   **B.** true   **C.** false   **D.** false   **E.** false

Neural tube defects are the result of a failure of closure of the neural tube during the third week of intrauterine life. The anti-epileptics sodium valproate and carbamazepine are associated with neural tube defects. There is increased alpha-fetoprotein in the amniotic fluid with a neural tube defect. Spina bifida occulta may be associated with neural tethering causing bladder and/or lower limb problems.

Exam 1

Answers

A 9. **A.** false **B.** true **C.** false **D.** false **E.** false

Lennox-Gastaut syndrome is an epilepsy syndrome comprising multiple seizure types and a characteristic EEG. There is developmental regression and the epilepsy is often intractable.

A 10. **A.** false **B.** false **C.** true **D.** true **E.** true

Other side-effects of phenytoin include gum hypertrophy and aplastic anaemia. Features of toxicity are ataxia, tremor, nystagmus and dysarthria. Peripheral retinal atrophy is a side-effect of vigabatrin.

A 11. **A.** false **B.** true **C.** false **D.** false **E.** true

Juvenile myoclonic epilepsy characteristically features generalized seizures of myoclonic jerks of the arms on awakening. The gene is on chromosome 6. Sodium valproate is effective.

A 12. **A.** true **B.** true **C.** true **D.** false **E.** true

A normal child should be able to draw a cross and hop by age 4 years. A normal child can manage some of their buttons by age 3 years, and all of their buttons by age 4 years. Both tying shoelaces and riding a bicycle are normally attained by age 5 years.

A 13. **A.** true **B.** true **C.** true **D.** true **E.** true

Iris coloboma is a notching of the iris usually in the inferolateral quadrant. There may be involvement of the retina and optic nerve.

A 14. **A.** true **B.** false **C.** false **D.** true **E.** false

Congenital rubella syndrome and Lowe's oculocerebrorenal syndrome can cause a small pupil. Fabry's disease is a cause of cataract in childhood.

A 15. **A.** true **B.** false **C.** false **D.** false **E.** true

At the p50 (there is 50% saturation of the haemoglobin), the surrounding partial pressure of oxygen is normally 27 mmHg. This can be altered by a number of factors including methaemoglobinaemia, cyanotic congenital heart disease and hypothermia (all causing the curve to shift to the left and therefore increasing the affinity of oxygen for haemoglobin). The oxygen saturation of mixed venous blood is 75%.

16. **A.** true **B.** true **C.** true **D.** false **E.** true

A mild thrombocytosis may be present. In addition the red cells are hypochromic and microcytic. There is decreased serum iron and ferritin and increased total iron-binding capacity (TIBC).

17. **A.** true **B.** true **C.** true **D.** false **E.** false

In both thalassaemia major and immune haemolytic anaemia the anaemia is the cause of the splenomegaly.

18. **A.** true **B.** false **C.** true **D.** false **E.** true

Both Hermansky-Pudlak syndrome and Bernard-Soulier syndrome are platelet function disorders in which the bleeding time is prolonged.

19. **A.** true **B.** false **C.** false **D.** true **E.** true

Von Willebrand's disease has a prolonged APTT and bleeding time, and normal prothrombin time. Haemophilia A and B have normal prothrombin time and bleeding time, but prolonged APTT. Bleeding time is prolonged with impaired platelet function and numbers and capillary function.

20. **A.** true **B.** false **C.** true **D.** true **E.** false

Hereditary angioneurotic oedema is due to C1 inhibitor deficiency. Chronic granulomatous disease is due to a defect in the oxygen reduction pathway in polymorphonuclear leucocytes.

21. **A.** false **B.** false **C.** true **D.** false **E.** true

Staphylococcal scalded skin syndrome is usually due to *Staphylococcus aureus* group II phage types 3A, 3C, 55 and 71. It presents with a febrile, unwell infant and is life-threatening due to sepsis and dehydration. Rapid treatment with antibiotics and supportive measures are necessary. The skin loss is intra-epidermal, which may be demonstrated on frozen section if the diagnosis is in doubt.

Exam 1

Answers

A 22. **A.** true   **B.** true   **C.** false   **D.** true   **E.** true

Galactosaemia is autosomal recessive, and there is an inability to metabolize both galactose and lactose (the latter is composed of glucose + galactose). It is managed with a lactose- and galactose-free diet. Dysarthria is a particular problem. Ovarian failure is present even with therapy.

A 23. **A.** true   **B.** true   **C.** true   **D.** false   **E.** false

Hartnup disease is a defect of neutral amino acid transport across the intestinal mucosa and the renal tubules. It results in tryptophan deficiency, which is an essential amino acid. Diagnosis is made by urine and plasma amino acid profile.

A 24. **A.** false   **B.** true   **C.** true   **D.** false   **E.** false

Medium Chain Acyl CoA Dehydrogenase Deficiency (MCADD) is one of the most common fatty acid oxidation defects. It is an autosomal recessive disorder, and between 1 in 40 and 1 in 80 of the UK population are asymptomatic carriers. Around 80–90% of affected individuals have the same genetic mutation. It usually present by age 2 years. The clinical features include hypoglycaemia, acute encephalopathy and sudden death. Initial diagnosis is on elevated octanoyl carnitine in the presence of normal carnitine levels on blood test and a characteristic urine organic acid profile. Definitive diagnosis confirming the mutation with molecular genetic studies, or enzyme studies of skin fibroblasts showing reduced MCAD activity can be done.

A 25. **A.** true   **B.** false   **C.** true   **D.** true   **E.** false

Normal portal pressure is only 7 mmHg. Caput medusae results in blood flow away from the umbilicus. Perivertebral and perispinal collaterals may occur and *in extremis* may cause signs of spinal compression. Factor V Leiden deficiency occurs in up to 10–15% of the Caucasian population and may result in hypercoagulation and hepatic or portal vein thromboses. As younger children rely in part on an increase in their heart rate to counter hypovolaemia secondary to potential haemorrhage from varices, beta-blockers are not recommended to decrease portal pressure as this protective mechanism may therefore be compromised.

Shepherd R. Chapter 11. In *Diseases of the Liver and Biliary System in Childhood*. Ed. Kelly D. Oxford: Blackwell Science, 1999.

A **26.** **A.** true **B.** false **C.** false **D.** true **E.** true

Inheritance of Hirschsprung's disease is polygenic, and the incidence is greater in males than in females. An increase in sympathetic activity is due to the absence of parasympathetic ganglions in the plexi of Auerbach and Meissner.

A **27.** **A.** true **B.** false **C.** false **D.** false **E.** true

Eye complications occur equally in both conditions. Sclerosing cholangitis, chronic active hepatitis, cirrhosis and pericholangitis are all more common in ulcerative colitis (UC).

Leichtner A, Jackson W, Grand D. Chapter 27. In *Pediatric Gastrointestinal Disease*. Ed. Walker A *et al*. St Louis: Mosby, 1996.

A **28.** **A.** true **B.** false **C.** false **D.** true **E.** false

If children with Alagille's syndrome, usually inherited as an autosomal dominant condition, and also called arteriohepatic dysplasia, require liver transplantation it is due to uncontrollable itching and poor quality of life rather than liver failure, which is not common. Zellweger's syndrome (cerebrohepatorenal syndrome) is an example of a peroxisomal disorder but this group does not include Alagille's syndrome. Features of Alagille's include progressive intrahepatic bile duct paucity; intense pruritus; typical facies with hypertelorism, deep-set eyes, long nose, broad forehead and small mandible; posterior embryotoxon of the eyes; peripheral pulmonary stenosis and Fallot's tetralogy; tubulointerstitial nephropathy; butterfly vertebrae; tuberous xanthomas and raised serum cholesterol. It occurs at an incidence of 1 in 100 000 live births. Gene mapping is now possible with a gene defect localized to chromosome 20p (gene termed *JAG1*) coding for a ligand of Notch 1, which is one of a member of four transmembrane proteins.

Roberts E. Chapter 2. In *Diseases of the Liver and Biliary System in Childhood*. Ed. Kelly D. Oxford: Blackwell Science, 1999.

A **29.** **A.** true   **B.** true   **C.** true   **D.** false   **E.** true

Plasma cholesterol reflects liver synthetic function, like serum albumin and coagulation state and, if it is low, this reflects worsening liver function and a poorer prognosis. Neurodevelopmental delay and other subtle symptoms such as problems at school or lethargy can reflect chronic hepatic encephalopathy. Spontaneous bacterial peritonitis should always be suspected in children with ascites, abdominal pain and fever. Paracentesis reveals cloudy fluid with a neutrophil count of >250 per mL. *Klebsiella*, *Escherichia coli* or *Streptococcus pneumoniae* predominate.

Shepherd R. Chapter 11. In *Diseases of the Liver and Biliary System in Childhood*. Ed. Kelly D. Oxford: Blackwell Science, 1999.

A **30.** **A.** false   **B.** false   **C.** true   **D.** false   **E.** true

Oxygenated blood is transported from the placenta to the fetus via the umbilical vein. The ductus venosus drains into the inferior vena cava.

A **31.** **A.** true   **B.** true   **C.** false   **D.** false   **E.** true

Chromosome 22q11 microdeletion is also associated with aortic arch anomalies.

A **32.** **A.** true   **B.** false   **C.** true   **D.** true   **E.** false

Torsades de Pointes may be congenital or acquired. The acquired form may be due to an electrolyte disturbance including hypomagnesaemia and hypocalcaemia, drugs including amiodarone and sotalol, organophosphate poisoning and low protein states including anorexia nervosa.

A **33.** **A.** false   **B.** false   **C.** true   **D.** true   **E.** true

The murmur of a ventricular septal defect (VSD) is pansystolic (though may be shorter if a small defect) and loudest at the lower left sternal edge. A loud P2 signals pulmonary hypertension is present.

A 34. A. false **B.** false **C.** true **D.** true **E.** true

Treatment with pacemaker insertion is only required if
there are symptoms or the daytime pulse rate is below
60 bpm in an infant. 15% of cases are secondary to structural
congenital heart disease including atrioventricular septal
defect. Maternal anti-Ro antibodies cause atrophy and
fibrosis of the AV node, and therefore result in complete heart
block.

A 35. A. false **B.** false **C.** false **D.** true **E.** true

The anion gap is the apparent disparity between the total
cation and the total anion concentration in the blood, which
occurs because some anions are not routinely measured. When
an acid load is present, the bicarbonate concentration falls
and this increases the anion gap. The normal anion gap is
10–12 mmol/L. In metabolic acidosis, it is dependent on chloride
concentration and may be normal or increased depending on
the cause of the acidosis. If the chloride is normal, the anion
gap is increased, and if the chloride is raised, the anion gap is
normal.

A 36. A. false **B.** true **C.** true **D.** true **E.** true

Fanconi's syndrome is a generalized defect in proximal renal
tubular function. It may be congenital (e.g. idiopathic,
galactosaemia, Wilson's disease, cystinosis, tyrosinaemia type 1)
or acquired (e.g. hyperparathyroidism, vitamin D deficiency,
various drugs, chemotherapy and glue-sniffing).

A 37. A. false **B.** false **C.** true **D.** false **E.** true

The haemolytic uraemic syndrome involves renal failure,
microangiopathic haemolytic anaemia and thrombocytopenia,
and can present with dangerous hyperkalaemia. Familial disease
has a worse prognosis.

A 38. A. true **B.** false **C.** true **D.** false **E.** false

Alport syndrome involves a hereditary nephritis,
sensorineural deafness and ocular defects (including
cataract).

A 39. **A.** false **B.** true **C.** true **D.** true **E.** true

Surfactant increases lung compliance at low lung volumes and decreases lung compliance at high lung volumes.

A 40. **A.** false **B.** true **C.** false **D.** true **E.** false

Cystic fibrosis is caused by a defect in the cystic fibrosis transmembrane regulator (*CFTR*) gene on chromosome 7. The CFTR protein is a chloride channel. Mutation results in abnormal chloride (and sodium) secretions, resulting in thick secretions high in sodium. The children may develop a hypokalaemic alkalosis due to sodium and potassium loss in sweat.

A 41. **A.** false **B.** false **C.** false **D.** false **E.** true

Oligoarticular juvenile idiopathic arthritis (JIA) is more common in girls and is rheumatoid factor negative. Approximately 20% of cases go on to affect more joints after 6 months (extended oligoarticular JIA). The ankles, knees and elbows are typically affected.

A 42. **A.** false **B.** false **C.** true **D.** true **E.** true

Inguinal hernias are usually indirect in children due to a patent processus vaginalis. They are more common in boys and on the right side.

A 43. **A.** false **B.** true **C.** false **D.** false **E.** true

Octreotide is a somatostatin analogue. It can cause a transient alopecia. It rarely causes altered liver function tests.

British National Formulary, 2007.

A 44. **A.** false **B.** true **C.** false **D.** true **E.** true

Mycophenolate mofetil is metabolized to the active mycophenolic acid. Gastrointestinal side-effects are common including abdominal discomfort, diarrhoea, nausea, vomiting and constipation. More severe side-effects include pancreatitis. It also causes bone marrow suppression. There is a higher risk of side-effects in children.

British National Formulary, 2005.

A 45. **A.** false **B.** true **C.** false **D.** false **E.** false

Doxorubicin commonly causes mucositis and more
rarely SVT related to administration of the drug. Cardiomyopathy
is seen at high cumulative doses (so total dose is limited).

British National Formulary, 2007.

A 46. **A.** false **B.** false **C.** false **D.** false **E.** false

Anorexia nervosa causes a hypochloraemic alkalosis (due to
vomiting), elevated growth hormone and rT3, and decreased T3,
LH and FSH.

A 47. **A.** false **B.** false **C.** true **D.** true **E.** false

The incidence of monozygotic twins is 3.5 in 1000 pregnancies.
There is a 1 in 66 spontaneous rate for dizygotic twins. Twin-twin
transfusion syndrome affects monochorionic twins (i.e. share the
same placenta).

A 48. **A.** true **B.** true **C.** true **D.** true **E.** true

Neonatal pulmonary haemorrhage is also associated with
coagulopathies.

A 49. **A.** true **B.** false **C.** false **D.** false **E.** true

Osteopenia of prematurity is classically seen in VLBW (very low
birth weight) premature infants and those with severe IUGR. It
may also be seen in infants with inadequate milk intake. Clinical
rickets is uncommon, though rib fractures in babies with chronic
lung disease may be seen. Calcium is normal, and alkaline
phosphatase and PTH are high.

A 50. **A.** true **B.** true **C.** true **D.** false **E.** false

Infants of mothers of black racial origin and those who smoke
have lower neonatal levels of bilirubin.

A 51. **A.** false **B.** true **C.** false **D.** true **E.** true

Preterm infants need approximately 120 kcal/kg/day, but sick
infants have a higher calorific requirement, up to 150 kcal/kg/day.

Glucose polymers are better absorbed than lactose in preterm infants because they have decreased intestinal lactase. Breast milk is 7% lactose compared with 4.8% for cow's milk.

A **52.** **A.** false **B.** true **C.** false **D.** true **E.** true

The syndrome of inappropriate antidiuretic hormone secretion (SIADH) tends to be asymptomatic until features of hyponatraemia and water intoxication develop. The clinical features are appetite loss, nausea, vomiting, confusion, irritability, personality change, fits and eventual coma. There is no evidence of dehydration, no oedema and normal blood pressure.

A **53.** **A.** false **B.** true **C.** false **D.** true **E.** false

Ultra-short acting insulin has an onset of 10 minutes, a peak action at 1 hour and a duration of 3–4 hours. Short-acting insulin has an onset of 30 minutes, peak action at 2 hours and a duration of 5–6 hours.

A **54.** **A.** false **B.** false **C.** true **D.** true **E.** false

Congenital hypothyroidism is usually sporadic. It is twice as common in females. It is usually detected via neonatal screening and if treated promptly, normal intelligence is possible. The IQ of the child directly relates to how rapidly treatment is commenced (prior to 6 weeks of age, average IQ = 100; 6 weeks to 3 months of age, average IQ = 95; 3 to 6 months of age, average IQ = 75). It is rarely associated with goitre.

A **55.** **A.** false **B.** false **C.** true **D.** true **E.** true

In congenital adrenal hyperplasia due to 21-hydroxylase deficiency, the preceding substance in the steroid hormone biosynthesis pathway – 17-OH-progesterone – is elevated. In addition blockade of the glucocorticoid pathway results in a reduction in the negative feedback effects of the glucocorticoids on the anterior pituitary gland causing ACTH elevation. The mineralocorticoid pathway and the glucocorticoid pathway (producing cortisol) are blocked. The steroid pathway is deflected down the androgenetic pathway, causing high testosterone and androstenedione.

A 56. **A.** false **B.** false **C.** false **D.** true **E.** false

Girls are usually diagnosed earlier than boys, as the most obvious clinical feature of the most common form (due to 21-hydroxylase deficiency) is ambiguous genitalia (in girls) due to androgen excess. The androgen excess does not cause any clearly abnormal appearance of the external genitalia in boys. They are a group of autosomal recessive disorders due to defects in the biosynthesis of cortisol. The late-onset form of 21-hydroxylase deficiency is uncommon and presents in pubertal girls with menstrual irregularity and hirsutism. 3-β-hydroxysteroid dehydrogenase deficiency is salt-wasting and does not cause hypertension.

A 57. **A.** false **B.** false **C.** false **D.** false **E.** true

Pertussis, influenza and typhoid are killed organism vaccines; diphtheria is a toxoid vaccine. The live attenuated vaccines include measles, mumps, rubella, varicella zoster virus, BCG, oral polio and yellow fever.

A 58. **A.** true **B.** true **C.** true **D.** true **E.** false

Giardiasis can cause acute diarrhoea with nausea and vomiting, and abdominal cramps and distension. Infection may, however, be asymptomatic resulting in a chronic carrier.

A 59. **A.** false **B.** false **C.** false **D.** false **E.** false

Mumps infection causes an initially unilateral, but within a few days bilateral, parotitis. Subclinical infection is contagious. Mumps infection is subclinical in about one-third of cases. It is most common in the winter and spring. The incubation period is long (2–3 weeks).

A 60. **A.** true **B.** true **C.** true **D.** true **E.** true

Roseola infantum (exanthem subitum) is associated with HHV-6 infection. It causes a sudden onset of high fever with associated generalized macular rash. It is thought to be the cause of up to one-third of febrile convulsions.

Q 1. The features of Treacher-Collins syndrome include

    A. Narrow airway
    B. Malar hyperplasia
    C. Severe malformation of external auricles
    D. Visual loss
    E. Conductive deafness

Q 2. In Williams syndrome

    A. Intelligence is normal
    B. Inheritance is X-linked dominant
    C. They have a friendly personality
    D. Dental defects may be seen
    E. Renal artery stenosis occurs

Q 3. In Klinefelter's syndrome

    A. Downward lens dislocation is seen
    B. The phenotype is tall and slim
    C. The karyotype is 47,XYY
    D. The penis and testes are of normal size in childhood
    E. Features are variable

Q 4. The following teratogens and effects are associated

    A. Isotretinoin – Hydrocephalus
    B. Carbamazepine – Neural tube defects
    C. Thalidomide – Ebstein's anomaly
    D. Warfarin – Nasal hypoplasia
    E. Phenytoin – Nail hypoplasia

Q 5. During the cell cycle

    A. DNA replication takes place during interphase
    B. Mitosis is the process of cytoplasmic division
    C. Haploid cell creation is known as meiosis

D. The length of the cycle varies in different cell types

E. During anaphase new nuclear membranes are formed around the two sets of chromosomes

Q 6. Regarding the spinal cord

A. Up to the third fetal month the cord extends the whole length of the vertebral canal

B. The filum terminale is attached to the second sacral vertebra

C. In the newborn the cord terminates at the upper border of the third lumbar vertebra

D. The spinothalamic tracts contain sensory fibres of fine touch and proprioception

E. The pyramidal tract contains motor fibres from the ipsilateral motor cortex

Q 7. Regarding the auditory (VIIIth) cranial nerve

A. Cochlear fibres terminate in the cochlear nuclei of the medulla from which efferent fibres ascend to the superior colliculus or the LGB

B. Temporal lobe tumours can give rise to visual hallucinations

C. The auditory cortex is located on the inferior temporal gyrus

D. Lesions of the cochlear division of the auditory nerve always result in deafness accompanied by tinnitus

E. Lesions of the vestibulocerebellar pathway result in ataxia

Q 8. Infantile spasms

A. Are usually of identifiable cause

B. May be extensor or flexor

C. Are more common in boys

D. Are associated with developmental arrest

E. May be caused by lissencephaly

Q 9. Benign rolandic epilepsy

A. Is most common at the age of 9–10 years

B. Is associated with a loss of language skills

C. Involves myoclonic 'drop' attacks

D. Shows a repetitive spike focus in the centrotemporal area

E. Responds to carbamazepine

Q 10. **The following are major diagnostic criteria for tuberous sclerosis**

    A. Retinal hamartomas (phakoma)
    B. Fibrous plaque of the forehead
    C. Lisch nodules in the iris
    D. Infantile spasms
    E. Pulmonary lymphangioleiomyomatosis

Q 11. **The Landau-Kleffner syndrome**

    A. Usually presents in infancy
    B. Is more common in girls
    C. Is autosomal recessive
    D. Is characterized by loss of fine motor skills
    E. EEG abnormalities are more common during sleep

Q 12. **A normal 9-month-old child can**

    A. Wave 'bye-bye'
    B. Use a pincer grasp
    C. Release objects
    D. Scribble
    E. Eat finger foods

Q 13. **Regarding aniridia**

    A. It may be associated with optic nerve hypoplasia
    B. It may be autosomal dominant
    C. If autosomal dominant, yearly abdominal ultrasound scans should be undertaken to screen for Wilms' tumour
    D. One-third of cases will develop Wilms' tumour
    E. It is associated with retinoblastoma

Q 14. **Bilateral cataract in childhood may be seen in association with**

    A. Alport syndrome
    B. Conradi's syndrome
    C. Anterior segment dysgenesis
    D. Aicardi's syndrome
    E. Hyperthyroidism

Q 15. **The following cause the oxyhaemoglobin dissociation curve to shift to the left**

    A. Acute acidosis
    B. Fever
    C. Methaemoglobin
    D. Carboxyhaemoglobin
    E. Sickle cell haemoglobin

Q 16. **The following can cause a macrocytic anaemia**

    A. Fanconi's anaemia
    B. Orotic aciduria
    C. Hyperthyroidism
    D. Down's syndrome
    E. Lead poisoning

Q 17. **Iron overload can cause**

    A. Cardiac failure
    B. Delayed puberty
    C. Osteoporosis
    D. Altered skin colour
    E. Hyperparathyroidism

Q 18. **In haemophilia A**

    A. 50% of cases are spontaneous mutations
    B. The gene is located on chromosome 10
    C. Intracerebral bleeds are relatively common
    D. Desmopressin may be used to treat mild disease
    E. Before major surgery, factor VIII levels of 70% of normal are aimed for

Q 19. **In a 1-year-old boy with eczema, recurrent chest infections and a low platelet count, the most likely diagnosis is**

    A. Hermansky-Pudlak syndrome
    B. Wiskott-Aldrich syndrome
    C. Glanzmann thrombasthenia
    D. Omenn's syndrome
    E. Bruton's disease

Q 20. **Regarding type IV hypersensitivity reactions**

   A. They are antibody-dependent cytotoxic reactions
   B. They can be transferred from one animal to another via serum
   C. Contact hypersensitivity is an example
   D. They can result in a granuloma
   E. Serum sickness is an example

Q 21. **The following conditions are associated with erythema nodosum**

   A. Behçet's syndrome
   B. Lymphosarcoma
   C. Measles
   D. Cat scratch disease
   E. Ulcerative colitis

Q 22. **Non-ketotic hyperglycinaemia**

   A. May present in the neonatal period
   B. Is autosomal dominant
   C. Is a cause of myoclonic seizures
   D. Causes osteoporosis
   E. Is seen in Down's syndrome

Q 23. **In hereditary fructose intolerance**

   A. There is an inability to metabolize fructose or sucrose
   B. Liver disease may occur
   C. Breast-feeding is contraindicated
   D. There is no effective treatment
   E. There is a urea cycle defect

Q 24. **The organic acidaemias**

   A. Show elevated plasma ketones during attacks
   B. Are a cause of renal impairment in the long term
   C. Are a cause of dysostosis multiplex
   D. Are managed with a low protein diet
   E. Include maple syrup urine disease

Q 25. **In acute liver failure**

   A. Aminotransferase levels are not predictive of the outcome
   B. Due to sodium valproate therapy the chance for a
       neurologically intact outcome is very poor

C. Hyperventilation usually accompanies stage II–III hepatic encephalopathy and may result in respiratory alkalosis
   D. Fluid restriction to <75% of maintenance is the key strategy in prevention of intracerebral oedema
   E. Coagulation support should only be used if active bleeding occurs or to cover invasive procedures

Q 26. **Biliary atresia is characterized by**

   A. An absence of a gallbladder on fasting ultrasound
   B. Biliary duct proliferation on liver biopsy
   C. Poor uptake of radioisotope into the liver after pre-administration of phenobarbitone for 5 days
   D. Facial dysmorphism with hypertelorism, deep-set eyes and a small mandible
   E. Conjugated hyperbilirubinaemia in the first 24 hours of life

Q 27. **In children with primary hepatic tumours**

   A. Hepatocellular carcinoma is commoner under the age of 4 years than hepatoblastoma
   B. Abdominal pain will be the presenting feature in 90%
   C. Jaundice occurs in less than 10%
   D. Plain abdominal X-ray will demonstrate calcification in 40–50% of hepatocellular carcinoma
   E. Hepatoblastoma has a well-established link with Beckwith-Wiedemann syndrome

Q 28. **In a child who appears to have malabsorption**

   A. Anti-endomyseal antibody is 99.5% sensitive for coeliac disease
   B. Faecal elastase is the most practically useful test for pancreatic insufficiency
   C. Giardiasis may be diagnosed by faecal examination in 70% of cases
   D. A small bowel biopsy is necessary for the diagnosis of abetalipoproteinaemia
   E. Primary lactase deficiency is a common cause

Q 29. **Regarding micronutrient and vitamin deficiencies**

   A. Dermatitis, dementia and diarrhoea occurs with a deficiency of niacin (or nicotinamide)

B. Symmetrical polyneuropathy occurs with thiamine deficiency

C. Raised S-T segments on the ECG can occur with vitamin A deficiency

D. Selenium deficiency occurs within 6 weeks of commencement of total parenteral nutrition

E. Vitamin A is found mainly in fish when a child is on a dairy-free diet

Q 30. The following are normal age-related vital signs

A. Neonatal respiratory rate – 40–60 per minute

B. Neonatal systolic blood pressure – above 95 mmHg

C. Pulse rate in a toddler of 2 years – 120 beats per minute

D. Respiratory rate in an infant of 18 months – 60 per minute

E. Pulse rate in a newborn – 60 beats per minute

Q 31. The following conditions are causes of cardiomegaly on chest X-ray

A. Ebstein's anomaly

B. Pericardial effusion

C. 22q11 deletion

D. Ventricular septal defect

E. Tetralogy of Fallot

Q 32. Dilated cardiomyopathy may be caused by

A. Doxorubicin

B. Iron overload

C. Carnitine deficiency

D. Diphtheria

E. Adriamycin

Q 33. Infective endocarditis

A. Causes erythema marginatum

B. Risk is higher in cardiac defects with low velocity flow

C. Is seen with ostium secundum atrial septal defects

D. May be chronic

E. Causes Roth spots

Q 34. Transposition of the great arteries

A. Presents with cyanosis after 3 days of life

B. Has a diastolic murmur

C. Has a normal ECG

D. Shows a 'coeur en sabot' appearance on chest X-ray

E. Is initially treated in an emergency with indomethacin

Q 35. Atrial natriuretic peptide has the following effects

A. Increased renin levels

B. Sodium retention

C. Increased glomerular filtration rate

D. Hypertension

E. Increased aldosterone levels

Q 36. Findings in proximal renal tubular acidosis are

A. Low serum bicarbonate

B. Urine pH above 5.5

C. Hyperkalaemia

D. Normal anion gap

E. Growth failure

Q 37. The following can cause proteinuria

A. Lymphoma

B. Fever

C. Exercise

D. Urinary tract infection

E. Standing upright for prolonged periods of time

Q 38. Henoch-Schonlein purpura

A. Most commonly affects teenagers

B. Is most common in the autumn

C. Can involve a destructive arthritis of the large joints

D. Causes an elevated serum IgA in most cases

E. May cause haemoptysis

Q 39. The following are true regarding the paediatric airway

A. The narrowest part of the trachea is at the cricoid

B. The occiput is larger than in adults

C. The glottis is located at C5 in neonates

D. The tongue is larger than in adults

E. Infants are obligate nasal breathers

Q 40. The following are causes of bronchiectasis

A. Measles
B. Inhaled foreign body
C. Asthma
D. Cystic fibrosis
E. Tuberculosis

Q 41. Regarding autoantibodies

A. Anti-ds DNA are specific for dermatomyositis
B. Anti-Jo-1 are seen in SLE
C. Anticentromere antibodies are present in CREST syndrome
D. Anti-Sm antibodies are present in the normal population
E. ANA positive disease in oligoarticular juvenile idiopathic arthritis is associated with a decreased risk of eye disease

Q 42. Intussusception

A. Is associated with Henoch-Schonlein purpura
B. Is successfully reduced by air or contrast enema in 50% of cases
C. Usually occurs just distal to the ileo-caecal valve
D. Is more common in females
E. Is associated with lymphoma

Q 43. Orlistat

A. Increases sensitivity to insulin at hepatic and peripheral levels
B. Should be given in conjunction with a low fat diet
C. May result in vitamin B deficiency
D. Can cause hypothyroidism
E. Is known to be effective in weight reduction in preschool children

Q 44. Erythropoietin

A. May cause hypertensive crises
B. Causes a dose-dependent thrombcytopenia
C. Can cause hypokalaemia
D. Can cause myoclonic seizures
E. May induce pure red cell aplasia

Q 45. **Hepatic first-pass metabolism can be avoided by giving a drug**

  A. Orally
  B. Sublingually
  C. Subcutaneously
  D. Rectally
  E. By intramuscular injection

Q 46. **The following would be consistent with features of autism in a 3-year-old boy**

  A. Echolalia
  B. Late development of number comprehension
  C. Interest in detail
  D. Good concentration
  E. Fascination with movement

Q 47. **In congenital cytomegalovirus infection**

  A. 75% of fetal infections are asymptomatic
  B. Up to 10% of affected infants develop neurological sequelae
  C. It is the most common congenital infection in the UK
  D. Periventricular cerebral calcifications are a feature
  E. Radiolucent bone lesions are seen

Q 48. **The following features are true of fetal development**

  A. Pupillary light reaction is consistently present from 26 weeks' gestation
  B. Leg buds appear in the sixth week of gestation
  C. Lactase is detectable from 20 weeks' gestation
  D. The fetal heart begins to beat in the fifth week of gestation
  E. The skull is the first fetal bone to ossify

Q 49. **The following are consistent with findings in a normal 32-week premature infant**

  A. The ear pinna springs back when folded
  B. Breast tissue appears
  C. The testes lie in the inguinal canal
  D. The soles of the feet are smooth
  E. The clitoris is covered by labia majora

Q 50. Causes of polycythaemia in newborns include

   A. Maternal diabetes
   B. Neonatal hypothyroidism
   C. Down's syndrome
   D. Pre-eclampsia
   E. Large for gestational age

Q 51. The following are features of neonatal vitamin E deficiency

   A. Haemolytic anaemia
   B. Thrombocytopenia
   C. Bone demineralization
   D. Hepatosplenomegaly
   E. Alopecia

Q 52. 1, 25-dihydroxycholecalciferol (calcitriol)

   A. Is synthesized in the liver
   B. Causes calcium uptake by the gut
   C. Stimulates bone resorption
   D. Is the main circulating vitamin D metabolite in the circulation
   E. Production is stimulated by hypophosphataemia

Q 53. The following are causes of persistent neonatal hypoglycaemia

   A. Hypopituitarism
   B. Fatty acid oxidation defects
   C. Intrauterine growth retardation
   D. Lysosomal storage disorders
   E. Galactosaemia

Q 54. The following are causes of hypocalcaemia

   A. Tuberculosis
   B. Thiazide diuretics
   C. Williams syndrome
   D. DiGeorge syndrome
   E. Vitamin A intoxication

Q 55. Causes of tall stature in childhood include

   A. Noonan syndrome
   B. Hypochondroplasia
   C. Pseudohypoparathyroidism

D. Homocystinuria

E. Obesity

Q 56. **Causes of short stature in childhood include**

A. Beckwith-Wiedemann syndrome

B. Hyperthyroidism

C. Pseudopseudohypoparathyroidism

D. Cranial irradiation

E. Prader-Willi syndrome

Q 57. **The combined DTaP/IPV/Hib vaccination**

A. May cause diarrhoea in the 24 hours post-vaccination

B. Is a cause of febrile convulsions

C. Should not be given to a child who has had anaphylaxis to streptomycin

D. Should not be given to a child who has had anaphylaxis to neomycin

E. Contains thiomersal

Q 58. **Parvovirus B19**

A. Does not harm the fetus in maternal infection

B. Manifests as a lacy rash on the trunk

C. May cause arthritis

D. May cause an aplastic crisis in a child with leukaemia

E. Is also known as erythema subitum

Q 59. **Regarding *Bordetella pertussis* infection**

A. It has an incubation of 14–21 days

B. It is a Gram-positive coccobacillus

C. It may cause rectal prolapse

D. Antibiotic therapy is not useful late in the disease

E. Mortality is usually due to secondary bacterial pneumonia

Q 60. **Herpangina**

A. Is an acute bacterial infection

B. Is an infection of the submandibular and sublingual spaces

C. Develops after dental extractions

D. Is characterized by central chest pain

E. Is characterized by pharyngeal vesicles

A 1. **A.** true **B.** false **C.** true **D.** true **E.** true

Children with Treacher-Collins syndrome have facial abnormalities of malar hypoplasia, downslanting palpebral fissures, lower lid defects and external ear malformation. Approximately one-third have visual loss, and almost 50% have conductive deafness. The narrow airway can make intubation difficult.

A 2. **A.** false **B.** false **C.** true **D.** true **E.** true

Williams syndrome is due to uniparental disomy, and is usually sporadically inherited. Intelligence is low with an IQ of around 55. Dental problems include partial adontia and enamel hypoplasia. Renal artery stenosis can cause hypertension. In addition, supravalvular aortic stenosis and peripheral pulmonary stenosis are described.

A 3. **A.** false **B.** true **C.** false **D.** false **E.** true

Klinefelter's syndrome has the karyotype 47,XXY. The testes and penis are small in childhood and remain so at adolescence, when there is partial virilization, and gynaecomastia occurs in about one-third of those affected. There is primary infertility.

A 4. **A.** true **B.** true **C.** true **D.** true **E.** true

A 5. **A.** true **B.** false **C.** true **D.** true **E.** false

Mitosis is the process of nuclear division, and cytokinesis that of cytoplasmic division. New nuclear membranes are formed around the two sets of chromosomes in telophase, the final stage of mitosis. During anaphase the centromeres of each chromosome split, separating the sister chromatids.

A 6. **A.** true **B.** false **C.** false **D.** false **E.** false

The spinal cord extends the whole length of the vertebral canal up to the third fetal month and then gradually becomes relatively shorter as the vertebrae grow faster, to terminate at the lower border of the third lumbar vertebrae in the newborn. The spinal cord tapers to the conus medullaris from which pia mater in a sheath of dura (the filum terminale) continues down and is attached to the coccyx. Sensory fibres of fine touch and proprioception are contained in the posterior columns, and the spinothalamic tracts contain the sensory fibres of pain and temperature. The motor fibres decussate in the medulla and hence are crossed in the pyramidal (motor) tract.

Anatomy for Anaesthetists. Ed. Ellis H & Feldman S, 6th edn 1993, Oxford: Blackwell Science, pp. 130–4.

A 7. **A.** false **B.** false **C.** false **D.** false **E.** true

The auditory (VIIIth) cranial nerve consists of both *cochlear* (concerned with hearing) and *vestibular* (concerned with equilibrium) fibres. The pathway of the cochlear fibres runs from the ganglion cells of the cochlea to the dorsal and ventral cochlear nuclei of the medulla where they terminate. Efferent fibres then run from these nuclei to the *inferior* colliculus or the *medial* geniculate body. Temporal lobe tumours may cause auditory hallucinations. The auditory cortex is on the superior temporal gyrus. Lesions of the cochlear division do not always result in tinnitus.

Anatomy for Anaesthetists. Ed. Ellis H & Feldman S, 6th edn 1993, Oxford: Blackwell Science, pp. 286–7.

A 8. **A.** true **B.** true **C.** true **D.** true **E.** true

Infantile spasms may be extensor, flexor or mixed seizures. The cause is known in around 80% of cases.

A 9. **A.** true **B.** false **C.** false **D.** true **E.** true

The centrotemporal area is known as the rolandic area. The seizures involve drooling or abnormal sensations around the mouth, and then secondary generalization.

A 10. **A.** true **B.** true **C.** false **D.** false **E.** true

Lisch nodules in the iris are seen in neurofibromatosis. The major diagnostic features of tuberous sclerosis are adenoma sebaceum or forehead plaque, ungual or periungual fibromas, shagreen patch, multiple retinal nodular hamartomas, cortical tuber, subependymal nodules, subependymal giant cell astocytoma, cardiac rhabdomyoma(s), pulmonary lymphangioleiomyomatosis and/or renal angiomyolipoma and hypomelanotic macules (ash-leaf macules). Infantile spasms are a clinical features, but not a diagnostic criteria.

A **11.** **A.** false **B.** false **C.** false **D.** false **E.** true

The Landau-Kleffner syndrome is of unknown aetiology. It is characterized by a loss of language skills, and seizures in up to 70% of cases. It is more common in boys and the average age of onset is 5 years.

A **12.** **A.** false **B.** true **C.** false **D.** false **E.** true

Waving 'bye-bye' and releasing objects should be attained by 1 year of age. Most children can scribble by 18 months. An infant can eat finger foods from about 6 months. The pincer grasp is present usually from 9 months, however it may not develop until 14 months in normal children.

A **13.** **A.** true **B.** true **C.** false **D.** false **E.** false

Aniridia may be sporadic or inherited as autosomal dominant. One-third of the sporadic cases will develop Wilms' tumour and therefore regular imaging should be done to screen for Wilms' tumour. It is associated with both optic nerve hypoplasia and nystagmus.

A **14.** **A.** true **B.** true **C.** true **D.** false **E.** false

Hyperparathyroidism causes bilateral cataract. Aicardi's syndrome may cause an iris coloboma.

A **15.** **A.** false **B.** false **C.** true **D.** true **E.** false

A shift in the oxyhaemoglobin dissociation curve to the left causes an increased affinity of haemoglobin for oxygen. Acute alkalosis, decreased temperature, carboxyhaemoglobin and methaemoglobin, and a fall in 2,3 DPG all cause the curve to shift to the left.

A 16. **A.** true **B.** true **C.** false **D.** true **E.** false

Hypothyroidism causes a macrocytic anaemia. Normal neonates have a macrocytosis due to the fetal haemoglobin. Lead poisoning can cause a sideroblastic (microcytic) anaemia.

A 17. **A.** true **B.** true **C.** true **D.** true **E.** false

The effects of iron overload may be divided into endocrine (growth failure, hypothyroidism, hypoparathyroidism, osteoporosis, insulin-dependent diabetes mellitus), skin (slate-grey colour), cardiac (cardiomyopathy causing arrythmias and cardiac failure) and liver (fibrosis, cirrhosis, hepatoma).

A 18. **A.** false **B.** false **C.** false **D.** true **E.** false

Around one-third of haemophilia A cases are spontaneous mutations, and the rest are of X-linked recessive inheritance (the gene being at chromosome Xq2.8). Intracerebral bleeds are rare. Prior to major surgery, factor VIII infusions are given aiming for normal levels (i.e. 100% of normal).

A 19. **A.** false **B.** true **C.** false **D.** false **E.** false

A 20. **A.** false **B.** false **C.** true **D.** true **E.** true

Type IV hypersensitivity reactions are delayed and involve cell-mediated immune reactions. There are three main types: contact hypersensitivity, tuberculin reaction and granulomatous reactions. Type IV hypersensitivity differs from other forms of hypersensitivity in that it cannot be transferred from one animal to another via serum.

A 21. **A.** true **B.** true **C.** true **D.** true **E.** true

There are many conditions that are associated with erythema nodosum, which may be sub-divided into infectious, gastrointestinal, iatrogenic, malignant and idiopathic.

A 22. **A.** true **B.** false **C.** true **D.** false **E.** false

Non-ketotic hyperglycinaemia can present in the neonatal period with seizures, lethargy, vomiting and coma. If survival occurs, severe mental retardation with myoclonic seizures and spasticity are seen. There is also a late-onset form. It is autosomal recessive.

A 23. **A.** true   **B.** true   **C.** false   **D.** false   **E.** false

Hereditary fructose intolerance is a disorder of carbohydrate metabolism, caused by a deficiency in aldolase B. Breast milk does not contain fructose. Treatment is by elimination of fructose from the diet.

A 24. **A.** true   **B.** true   **C.** false   **D.** true   **E.** false

The organic acidaemias include methylmalonic acidaemia and are characterized by neonatal or later intermittent attacks of vomiting, lethargy and severe ketoacidosis during intercurrent illnesses. During an episode, the blood glucose is low and ketones and ammonia are high. In the long term, renal impairment, mental retardation, movement disorders and faltering growth occur if untreated. Maple syrup urine disease is an aminoacidopathy.

A 25. **A.** true   **B.** true   **C.** true   **D.** true   **E.** true

A drop in ALT/AST (SGOT/SGPT) can reflect massive hepatocellular necrosis and little residual viable liver tissue. A mitochondria cytopathy uncovered by sodium valproate is usually responsible for fulminant liver failure in this instance and therefore multisystem (including neurological) involvement precludes survival even with liver transplant in nearly all cases. Metabolic acidosis may occur, but respiratory alkalosis also occurs in stage II–III encephalopathy. Coagulation is a good indicator of liver function and should not be artificially supported unless necessary. Vitamin K and the liver's response to it may yield useful information.

A 26. **A.** true   **B.** true   **C.** false   **D.** false   **E.** false

Liver biopsy usually distinguishes between neonatal hepatitis and biliary atresia but the two can still present with similar histological hepatic features – biliary duct hyperplasia is usually seen in biliary atresia and giant cells are typical of neonatal hepatitis. Phenobarbitone pre-administration prior to a liver isotope scan increases the likelihood of hepatobiliary excretion in neonatal hepatitis but not biliary atresia: it has no effect on uptake in either condition. If facial dysmorphism is seen with so-called 'pinched facies' of hypertelorism, deep-set eyes, small mandible and a long nose then arteriohepatic dysplasia, or Alagille's syndrome, should be suspected in the presence of jaundice. Biliary atresia is not characterized by jaundice in the first day of life as this is much more likely to be due to a haemolytic cause.

Davenport M, Howard E. Chapter 15. In *Diseases of the Liver and Biliary System in Childhood*. Ed. Kelly D. Oxford: Blackwell Science, 1999.

A **27.** **A.** false **B.** false **C.** true **D.** false **E.** true

Most hepatoblastomas occur under 18 months of age and hepatocellular carcinoma (HCC) is more common in older children. The short arm of chromosome 11 is implicated in the genetic aetiology of hepatoblastoma, and is associated with other embryonal tumours such as Wilms'. Conversely, HCC seems to be associated with environmental factors. An abdominal mass will be present in 50–60% of HCCs and 70% of hepatoblastomas, but pain only occurs in 10–20%. Weight loss and anorexia are similarly uncommon (20%), and jaundice only appears in 7–10% of cases. MRI is the investigation of choice with further imaging of the vascularity by hepatic angiography if required. Calcification is not a feature.

Morland B, Buckels J. Chapter 16. In *Diseases of the Liver and Biliary System in Childhood*. Ed. Kelly D. Oxford: Blackwell Science, 1999.

A **28.** **A.** false **B.** true **C.** false **D.** true **E.** false

Anti-endomyseal antibody is an IgA and as 1–4% of the general population have low IgA there may be a false negative result in these individuals. A maximum pick-up rate of *Giardia* in the stools of 20% can be expected, and hence a trial of metronidazole for 5–7 days may be a better diagnostic tool. Primary lactase deficiency is rare whereas post-gastroenteritis, secondary lactase deficiency is not uncommon. Late-onset congenital lactase deficiency occurs around the age of 10–14 years, especially in those of Mediterranean origin.

A **29.** **A.** true   **B.** true   **C.** false   **D.** false   **E.** false

Selenium stores are sufficient to account for requirements for 6 months when on a selenium-free diet (modern total parenteral nutrition (TPN) will have selenium added to it), and deficiency can cause cardiomyopathy, not pericarditis. Eggs, liver and green vegetables are good sources of vitamin A.

A **30.** **A.** true   **B.** false   **C.** true   **D.** false   **E.** false

The vital signs are very variable both between infants and in the same infant. A normal newborn has a respiratory rate of up to 60 per minute, systolic blood pressure is below 95 mmHg, and the pulse rate is above 120 beats per minute. A 2-year-old has a heart rate of 90–140 beats per minute, and the respiratory rate in an 18-month-old is 24–40 per minute.

A **31.** **A.** true   **B.** true   **C.** false   **D.** true   **E.** false

Tetralogy of Fallot causes a small 'coeur en sabot' appearance on chest X-ray.

A **32.** **A.** true   **B.** true   **C.** true   **D.** true   **E.** true

There are many causes of dilated cardiomyopathy, which may be broadly divided into genetic diseases, infections, nutritional causes and toxins.

A **33.** **A.** false   **B.** false   **C.** false   **D.** true   **E.** true

Erythema marginatum is seen in rheumatic fever. Infective endocarditis may be either acute or chronic. It is seen in particular with abnormal heart valves, but not with ostium secundum atrial septal defects. The risk is higher in high velocity flow defects. Roth spots are associated retinal haemorrhages.

A **34.** **A.** false   **B.** false   **C.** true   **D.** false   **E.** false

Transposition of the great arteries presents with cyanosis within hours of birth. There is no murmur, and the ECG is normal. The chest X-ray has a narrow upper mediastinum ('egg on side'). Emergency treatment is with prostaglandin infusion to keep the ductus arteriosus patent.

A. false **B.** false **C.** true **D.** false **E.** false

Atrial natriuretic peptides are secreted from the cardiac atria in response to increased stretch, increased osmolality and increased pressure. They cause a fall in renin and aldosterone levels, sodium excretion and a fall in blood pressure.

A 36. **A.** true **B.** false **C.** false **D.** true **E.** true

Proximal renal tubular acidosis is due to a failure of proximal tubular bicarbonate reabsorption. The serum bicarbonate, potassium and chloride are all low. Because the distal tubular acidification mechanisms are intact, the urine can be acidified (pH <5.5) when there is acidosis.

A 37. **A.** true **B.** true **C.** true **D.** true **E.** true

There are many causes of proteinuria, which can be divided into physiological and pathological. The physiological causes are orthostatic (standing upright for prolonged periods of time), exercise-induced and febrile proteinuria. Pathological causes can be divided into tubular disease, glomerular disease and other causes (e.g. urinary tract infection and lymphoma).

A 38. **A.** false **B.** false **C.** false **D.** true **E.** true

Henoch-Schönlein purpura is a vasculitis of small blood vessels, often following an upper respiratory tract infection. It most commonly affects children between age 3 and 10 years, and is more common in boys and in the late winter and early summer. The classical features are a rash, joint involvement, abdominal pain and haematuria. The arthritis is non-destructive. The serum IgA is elevated in over 50% of cases.

A 39. **A.** true **B.** true **C.** false **D.** true **E.** true

The glottis is at C3–4 in neonates and at C5 in adults.

A 40. **A.** true **B.** true **C.** false **D.** true **E.** true

A 41. **A.** false **B.** false **C.** true **D.** true **E.** false

Anti-ds DNA are specific for systemic lupus erythematosus. Anti-Jo-1 antibodies are seen in juvenile dermatomyositis. ANA positive disease in oligoarticular juvenile idiopathic arthritis is associated with an increased risk of eye disease.

A 42. **A.** true **B.** false **C.** false **D.** false **E.** true

Intussusception is an invagination of a distal segment of bowel into an adjacent proximal segment. It usually occurs just proximal to the ileo-caecal valve. It is more common in males. Air or contrast enema reduction is successful in about 75% of cases and is operator-dependent.

A 43. **A.** false **B.** true **C.** false **D.** false **E.** false

Orlistat reduces intestinal fat absorption and a low fat diet should be adhered to to reduce the side-effect of steatorrhoea. It can cause deficiency of the fat soluble vitamins (A, D, E and K) and these are therefore given as supplements. Studies are currently being undertaken in adolescents.

Viner R, Nicholls D. Managing obesity in secondary care: a personal practice. *Arch Dis Childhood*, 2005; **90** (4): 385–90.

A 44. **A.** true **B.** false **C.** false **D.** false **E.** true

Erythropoietin causes a dose-dependent thrombocytosis and can cause hyperkalaemia. Generalized tonic-clonic seizures can occur as part of a hypertensive crisis.

A 45. **A.** false **B.** true **C.** true **D.** false **E.** true

The hepatic first-pass effect is avoided if the drug does not enter the hepatic portal circulation. Hence, giving a drug transdermally or parenterally (IV, IM, SC) will avoid the effect. Some of the drug will enter the portal circulation when given rectally.

A 46. **A.** true **B.** false **C.** true **D.** false **E.** true

Features of autism include echolalia and speech delay, early development of numbers, an interest in detail, a fascination with movement, difficulty in moving from one activity to the next and a poor concentration span. In addition, they have limited eye contact and the child may relate to parts of a person rather than the whole person.

A 47. **A.** false **B.** true **C.** true **D.** true **E.** false

Congenital CMV infection is asymptomatic in 50% of cases. Around 5% present at birth and others present later. Deafness, which may be progressive, is the most prominent neurological sequelae. Radiolucent bone lesions are seen in congenital rubella syndrome.

A 48. **A.** false **B.** false **C.** false **D.** false **E.** false

The pupillary light reaction is consistently present from 32 weeks' gestation. The arm buds and leg buds appear in the fourth week of gestation. Lactase is not detectable until 28–30 weeks' gestation. The fetal heart begins to beat in the third week of gestation. The clavicle is the first fetal bone to ossify.

A 49. **A.** false **B.** false **C.** true **D.** false **E.** false

In a 32-week premature infant the ear pinna is soft and does not spring back when folded, there is no breast tissue (this appears from 36 weeks), there are one to two anterior plantar creases, and the clitoris is prominent and not covered by the labia majora.

A 50. **A.** true **B.** true **C.** true **D.** true **E.** false

Intrauterine hypoxia results in fetal polycythaemia. Causes of this include pre-eclampsia, intrauterine growth retardation and maternal smoking.

A 51. **A.** true **B.** false **C.** false **D.** false **E.** false

Vitamin E is necessary for stabilizing the red cell membrane. Deficiency causes a mild haemolytic anaemia with peripheral oedema and thrombocytosis.

A 52. **A.** false **B.** true **C.** true **D.** false **E.** true

1, 25-dihydroxycholecalciferol (calcitriol) is synthesized in the kidneys. Its production is stimulated by hypophosphataemia and PTH. It promotes both bone resorption and mineralization, as well as intestinal calcium and phosphate absorption. 25-hydroxycholecalciferol is the main circulating vitamin D metabolite.

A **53.** **A.** true   **B.** true   **C.** false   **D.** false   **E.** true

Intrauterine growth retardation causes a transient neonatal hypoglycaemia.

A **54.** **A.** false   **B.** false   **C.** false   **D.** true   **E.** false

Tuberculosis, thiazide diuretics, vitamin A intoxication and Williams syndrome are all causes of hypercalcaemia.

A **55.** **A.** false   **B.** false   **C.** false   **D.** true   **E.** true

Noonan syndrome and pseudohypoparathyroidism cause short stature. Hypochondroplasia is a skeletal dysplasia that also causes short stature. Obesity does result in tall stature during childhood, but eventual adult height is as predicted for parental heights.

A **56.** **A.** false   **B.** false   **C.** true   **D.** true   **E.** true

Cranial irradiation can cause damage to the hypothalamic-pituitary axis causing growth hormone deficiency. Beckwith-Wiedemann syndrome and hyperthyroidism both cause tall stature.

A **57.** **A.** true   **B.** true   **C.** true   **D.** true   **E.** false

The combined DTaP/IPV/Hib vaccination is contraindicated in infants who have had a previous anaphylaxis to neomycin, streptomycin or polymyxin B. In the 24 hours after vaccination there may be a mild increase in temperature, irritability and/or diarrhoea. Rarely, it may result in a febrile convulsion. This combined vaccine does not contain thiomersal.

A **58.** **A.** false   **B.** true   **C.** true   **D.** true   **E.** false

Parvovirus B19 can cause erythema infectiosum (fifth disease). This presents with red cheeks (slapped cheek disease) and a fine lacy rash on the body. Arthritis and arthralgia may appear as complications or the only symptom of parvovirus infection and are more common in adults. Congenital infection can cause hydrops fetalis and death, though most infected fetuses survive. Aplastic crises can be precipitated in infection in immunocompromised children and those with chronic haemolytic anaemias (e.g. sickle cell disease).

A. false   **B.** false   **C.** true   **D.** false   **E.** true

Bordetella pertussis is a Gram-negative coccobacillus. The incubation period is 7–14 days. Antibiotic therapy late in the disease does not decrease the severity of symptoms, but eliminates nasopharyngeal carriage of the organism.

A. false   **B.** false   **C.** false   **D.** false   **E.** true

Herpangina is a viral infection with usually Coxsackie A and B or echoviruses. There is a fever and vesicular rash and ulcers on the pharynx and buccal mucosa. Ludwig's angina is a bacterial cellulitis in the mouth occurring after dental extractions or mouth injury.

Exam 2

Answers

Q 1. The following conditions are autosomal recessive

A. Phenylketonuria
B. Polyposis coli
C. Noonan syndrome
D. Friedreich's ataxia
E. Congenital adrenal hyperplasia

Q 2. In Trisomy 18 the following may be seen

A. An association with older maternal age
B. Holoproscencephaly
C. Tetralogy of Fallot
D. Positional talipes
E. Micrognathia

Q 3. Cri du chat syndrome

A. Is due to partial deletion of the long arm of chromosome 5
B. Is incompatible with survival
C. May have normal intelligence
D. Includes macrocephaly
E. Has a single palmar crease

Q 4. Regarding the inheritance of Trisomy 21

A. Mosaicism accounts for around 5% of cases
B. The clinical features are milder in mosaicism
C. Robertsonian translocation accounts for about 20% of cases
D. The risk of recurrence is 100% if a parent has the translocation 21:21
E. The risk of recurrence is 25% if the father is a translocation carrier

Q 5. **The following disorders and mutations are correctly linked**

    A. Charcot-Marie-Tooth – Whole gene duplication
    B. Cystic fibrosis – Base pair insertion
    C. Duchenne muscular dystrophy – Missense mutation
    D. Sickle cell anaemia – Expanded tandem repeats
    E. Hb Bart's – Deletion or abnormality of all four alpha-globin genes

Q 6. **Regarding the facial nerve**

    A. The upper part of the motor nucleus of the facial nerve receives both crossed and uncrossed cortical fibres
    B. The geniculate ganglion contains fibres transmitting taste
    C. It transmits taste fibres from the posterior two-thirds of the tongue via the chorda tympani
    D. It conveys secretomotor fibres to the parotid gland
    E. It is purely motor in function once it emerges from the stylomastoid foramen

Q 7. **The occulomotor (IIIrd) cranial nerve**

    A. Conveys the sympathetic fibres for the ciliary muscle
    B. Supplies all the extrinsic eye muscles except inferior oblique
    C. Complete division results in double vision
    D. Complete division results in a divergent squint
    E. Runs in the lateral wall of the cavernous sinus

Q 8. **A meningomyelocele**

    A. Is a protrusion of the meninges only through a vertebral defect
    B. Is usually associated with sensory loss in the legs
    C. Is a cause of talipes
    D. Is a cause of slipped upper femoral epiphysis
    E. Is associated with hydrocephalus

Q 9. **Agenesis of the corpus callosum**

    A. May be inherited in X-linked recessive fashion
    B. Is associated with severe intellectual impairment
    C. Is seen in Trisomy 18
    D. May be asymptomatic
    E. Is seen in Aicardi's syndrome

Q 10. Childhood absence epilepsy

A. Is often associated with a positive family history
B. May include both typical and atypical absence seizures
C. Onset is usually in teenage years
D. Is more common in boys
E. Seizures may be induced by emotion

Q 11. Sodium valproate

A. Is the drug of choice in typical absence seizures
B. Causes hyperphagia
C. Has a dose-dependent association with thrombocytopenia
D. Is first-line therapy in complex partial seizures
E. Can cause transient elevation of liver enzymes

Q 12. The following reflexes and postural responses disappear at the described ages

A. Forward parachute – 9 months
B. Lateral propping reflex – 1 year
C. Palmar grasp – 2 months
D. Stepping reflex – 6 months
E. Moro reflex – 4 months

Q 13. The following conditions can cause corneal opacities

A. Infantile glaucoma
B. Dermoid
C. Congenital hereditary endothelial dystrophy
D. Dystichiasis
E. Telecanthus

Q 14. The following conditions can cause leucocoria

A. Buphthalmos
B. Colobomas
C. Coats' disease
D. Retinal detachment
E. Galactosaemia

Q 15. The following are true regarding haemoglobin

A. Fetal blood is composed of HbF and HbA
B. Haemopoeisis occurs initially in the yolk sac in the fetus

C. In the last trimester of fetal life haemopoeisis takes place in the bone marrow

D. HbA2 is composed of α 2–δ 2 polypeptide chains

E. HbF is composed of δ 2–γ 2 polypeptide chains

Q 16. **The following are causes of B12 deficiency in children**

    A. Crohn's disease

    B. Intestinal tuberculosis

    C. Trimethoprim

    D. Phenytoin

    E. Fish tapeworm

Q 17. **The following are true of hereditary spherocytosis**

    A. It may present with neonatal jaundice

    B. The anaemia may be mild

    C. The reticulocyte count is normal

    D. It can present at various ages

    E. Parvovirus infection can precipitate an aplastic crisis

Q 18. **In a child 3 months post-splenectomy the blood film would show**

    A. Target cells

    B. Monocytosis

    C. Pappenheimer granules

    D. Low platelet count

    E. Prickle cells

Q 19. **In a 5-year-old boy presenting with bruising and mucosal petechiae, and a platelet count of $25 \times 10^5/mm^3$, 10 days after chicken pox infection the most likely diagnosis is**

    A. Von Willebrand's disease

    B. Haemolytic anaemia

    C. Megaloblastic anaemia

    D. Acute idiopathic thrombocytopenic purpura

    E. Acute lymphoblastic leukaemia

Q 20. **Regarding polymorphonuclear granulocytes**

    A. They live for 2–3 weeks

    B. They are a type of antigen-presenting cell

C. They make up about 30% of the total normal blood leucocytes
D. They employ phagocytosis
E. They are antigen-specific

Q 21. Urticaria pigmentosa

A. Is a disorder involving a proliferation of eosinophils
B. Is a form of mastocytosis
C. Usually requires treatment
D. May resolve spontaneously
E. May cause abdominal pain

Q 22. Phenylketonuria

A. May cause severe vomiting in infancy
B. May cause seborrhoeic dermatitis
C. Is treated by excluding phenylalanine
D. If untreated during pregnancy can cause fetal abnormalities
E. Is classically associated with a fishy smell

Q 23. Homocystinuria

A. Is autosomal recessive
B. Is a urea cycle defect
C. Is due to cystathione synthase deficiency
D. May respond to pyridoxine therapy
E. Causes thromboembolism

Q 24. In Wilson's disease

A. There are increased copper levels in many tissues
B. Cirrhosis is a feature
C. Aplastic anaemia is a feature
D. It is a glycogen storage disorder
E. Screening of relatives is not possible

Q 25. Schwachman-Diamond syndrome

A. Can involve red cell aplasia
B. Can reveal a high HbF on electrophoresis
C. Can involve epiphyseal dysostosis
D. Progression to myeloid arrest can occur
E. Average survival is approximately 15 years

If a polyp or polyps are present in the colon of a 12-year-old boy

    A. Painful bright red bleeding with autolysis is the most common presentation

    B. Retinal pigmentation is an early clinical marker for familial adenomatous polyposis coli

    C. Mucosal pigmentation around the mouth indicates that there is a 50% chance of him developing malignant tumours outside the GI tract

    D. And are seen by barium follow through, then ulcerative colitis is a possible diagnosis

    E. Recurrent volvulus is likely after 1 year if removal is not undertaken

Q 27. **In children with diseases affecting the oral cavity**

    A. Swelling of the lips may be the sole manifestation of Crohn's disease

    B. Oral ulceration can be demonstrated in 60% of those with Behçet's disease

    C. Recurrent aphthous ulceration is usually due to cyclical neutropenia

    D. Ulcers due to tuberculosis are in most cases secondary to pulmonary disease

    E. Gum hypertrophy may be a manifestation of acrodermatitis enteropathica

Q 28. **In conjugated hyperbilirubinaemia in infancy**

    A. Choledochal cysts are the second commonest surgical cause

    B. Due to biliary atresia, a rapid rise in urobilinogen is seen on the first day

    C. Due to tyrosinaemia, urinary succinylacetone is a reliable diagnostic tool

    D. Due to alpha-1-antitrypsin deficiency, liver involvement is commonly accompanied by intrauterine growth retardation

    E. Kasai protoenterostomy is not effective for intrahepatic biliary atresia even if performed before 60 days of age

Q 29. **In a child or adolescent diagnosed with Wilson's disease**

    A. Acute psychosis may be the only presenting feature

    B. 24-hour copper excretion is markedly reduced after administration of penicillamine

Exam 3

Questions

C. All first-degree family members should be screened for pre-symptomatic disease

D. There is a 72% chance of association with HLA-A3

E. Penicillamine is the treatment of choice

Q 30. **In children**

A. The cardiac axis is left and anterior in the neonate

B. Normal splitting of the second heart sound on expiration is audible

C. A third heart sound can be normal

D. Stroke volume can be varied more than heart rate

E. A fourth heart sound can be normal

Q 31. **The following are causes of a right-sided aortic arch**

A. Truncus arteriosus

B. Dilated cardiomyopathy

C. Total anomalous pulmonary venous drainage

D. Ebstein's anomaly

E. Congenital vascular ring

Q 32. **The following conditions will result in a right thoracotomy scar**

A. Pulmonary artery band

B. Coarctation of the aorta repair

C. Blalock-Taussig shunt

D. Patent ductus arteriosus ligation

E. Atrial septal defect repair

Q 33. **Pulmonary atresia with a ventricular septal defect**

A. Is always duct-dependent

B. Causes a right-sided aortic arch on chest X-ray

C. Needs emergency treatment with prostaglandin E2

D. Has a single second heart sound

E. Is associated with Klinefelter's syndrome

Q 34. **In tetralogy of Fallot**

A. There is a pansystolic murmur

B. It may present with a murmur at 3 months of age

C. Corrective surgery is usually performed by age 1 year

D. Propranolol can be used to treat hypercyanotic spells

E. There is a single second heart sound

Q 35. **The following are predominantly reabsorbed in the distal renal tubule**

A. Water

B. Amino acids

C. Glucose

D. Galactose

E. Fructose

Q 36. **Features of distal renal tubular acidosis are**

A. Hypercalciuria

B. Osteomalacia

C. Low serum chloride

D. Nephrocalcinosis

E. Hypercalcaemia

Q 37. **In minimal change nephrotic syndrome**

A. There is an equal sex ratio

B. Urine has an albumin:creatinine ratio of <200 mg/mmol

C. Frothy urine is usually present

D. C3 is decreased

E. Red cell casts are present in the urine

Q 38. **In Fanconi's syndrome**

A. There is a generalized defect in distal renal tubular function

B. There is photophobia

C. There is a hypochloraemic metabolic acidosis

D. The anion gap is normal

E. There is increased urine bicarbonate loss

Q 39. **The respiratory system of a child compared to that of an adult**

A. Has a decreased compliance

B. Has decreased elastin

C. Has decreased airway resistance

D. Has more horizontal ribs

E. Has smaller alveoli

Q 40. In acute laryngo-tracheo-bronchitis (croup)

    A. Steroid nebulizers are ineffective
    B. Adrenaline causes sustained improvement
    C. There is usually little constitutional disturbance
    D. It is most common in infants under 1 year
    E. Arterial blood gas measurement is helpful in assessing severity

Q 41. Regarding systemic lupus erythematosus (SLE)

    A. Anti-nRNP is positive in 100% of cases
    B. Neonatal congenital heart block in infants of mothers with SLE is prevented by antenatal steroids
    C. Rheumatoid factor is positive in 50% of cases
    D. C3 is decreased in active disease
    E. Gottron's papules are seen on the knuckles

Q 42. Congenital diaphragmatic hernia is associated with

    A. Brachmann-de Lange syndrome
    B. Trisomy 18
    C. Down's syndrome
    D. Marfan syndrome
    E. Sotos syndrome

Q 43. The following are characteristic of first-order kinetics

    A. The enzyme responsible for the reaction is saturated
    B. The reaction is represented by a linear relationship
    C. The rate of elimination and elimination half-life is constant, irrespective of plasma concentration
    D. A constant proportion of drug is metabolized in a given time period
    E. The absolute amount eliminated is greatest when plasma concentration is greatest

Q 44. Tacrolimus

    A. Is a GABA inhibitor
    B. May cause cardiomyopathy
    C. Is less nephrotoxic than ciclosporin
    D. Is neurotoxic
    E. Can cause hallucinations

Q 45. Regarding desferioxamine

   A. It is given intradermally over 8–12 hours for iron overload
   B. Iron excretion is enhanced by administration of vitamin D
   C. It may be used to treat aluminium overload
   D. It can cause hypertension if given rapidly
   E. It can cause retinopathy

Q 46. Regarding autism

   A. An organic cause is found in around 30% of cases
   B. Siblings have a 10% prevalence of autism
   C. Monozygotic twin concordance is 25%
   D. There is an increased risk of epilepsy in teenage years
   E. Developmental stasis or regression is seen in 10% of cases at 15–18 months of age

Q 47. Hydrops fetalis may be caused by intrauterine infection with

   A. *Listeria monocytogenes*
   B. *Haemophilus influenzae*
   C. Cytomegalovirus
   D. *Treponema pallidum*
   E. Parvovirus B19

Q 48. Regarding congenital toxoplasmosis infection

   A. The risk of infant infection is greatest under 12 weeks' gestational age
   B. The risk of infant infection during the second trimester is 10%
   C. It may be acquired from soft cheeses
   D. Diffusely scattered cerebral calcification is seen
   E. Cardiac defects are a prominent feature of fetal infection

Q 49. Regarding neonatal Group B beta-haemolytic Streptococcal infection

   A. Approximately 10% of women have vaginal colonization with Group B β-haemolytic streptococci
   B. Only 25% of infants colonized during delivery develop sepsis
   C. Colonized infants born to mothers with premature rupture of membranes are at greater risk of sepsis

D. Colonized infants born to pyrexial mothers are at greater risk of sepsis

E. Neonatal Group B β-haemolytic Streptococcal infection may cause a late onset meningitis at 5–7 days

Q 50. Intrauterine growth retardation is associated with

A. Meconium aspiration
B. Polycythaemia
C. Perinatal asphyxia
D. Behavioural problems
E. Hypercalcaemia

Q 51. Colostrum differs from mature human breast milk in that it is

A. Lower in phospholipid
B. Higher in cholesterol
C. Lower in protein concentration
D. Higher in lactose
E. Higher in total fat composition

Q 52. The adrenal medulla secretes

A. Angiotensin II
B. Noradrenaline
C. Dehydroepiandrosterone
D. Aldosterone
E. Cortisol

Q 53. The following features would support a diagnosis of diabetes insipidus

A. Excessive perspiration
B. Failure to thrive
C. Intermittent low-grade fever
D. Glycosuria
E. New onset of nocturnal enuresis

Q 54. Multiple endocrine neoplasia (MEN) type I is characterized by

A. Parathyroid adenomas
B. Phaeochromocytoma
C. Mucosal neuromas

D. Medullary thyroid carcinoma

E. Mucocutaneous candidiasis

Q 55. Recognized findings in normal puberty include

A. Age of onset in girls is usually between 9 and 12 years

B. First sign in boys is enlargement of the penis

C. Diffuse thyroid enlargement

D. Menstruation usually commences at breast stage 3

E. First sign in girls is thelarche

Q 56. The following are features of McCune-Albright syndrome

A. Advanced bone age

B. Intracranial calcification

C. Ash-leaf macules

D. Adrenal gland hyperactivity

E. Ovarian gland hyperactivity

Q 57. Tetanus vaccine

A. Cannot be given to children with hypogammaglobulinaemia

B. Is contraindicated if there is a history of inflammatory bowel disease

C. After the primary course, should be boosted every 10 years

D. Is contraindicated in infants undergoing chemotherapy

E. Is an egg protein vaccine

Q 58. Concerning congenital syphilis

A. Syphilis infection during pregnancy has a transmission of 40%

B. When treated with penicillin there is no risk of the Jarisch-Herxheimer reaction

C. Causes destruction of the nasal bone and cartilage

D. May cause blindness

E. It causes a thrombocythaemia

Q 59. Scarlet fever

A. May present with abdominal pain and vomiting

B. Is associated with a grey-white tonsillar exudate

C. Causes conjunctival inflammation

D. Is characterized by perioral pallor

E. Is caused by Group B *Streptococcus*

Q **60.** **In *Mycoplasma pneumoniae* infection**

A. Up to 20% of children will have a pleural effusion

B. Approximately 25% of affected individuals produce cold agglutinins

C. The chest X-ray often looks unexpectedly mild

D. Sinusitis may occur

E. It can be isolated from the respiratory tract for months after infection and therefore provide a risk of spread to other family members

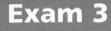
A 1. **A.** true **B.** false **C.** false **D.** true **E.** true

Both Polyposis coli and Noonan syndrome are autosomal dominant disorders.

A 2. **A.** true **B.** false **C.** true **D.** false **E.** true

Trisomy 18 (Edwards syndrome) is most likely to occur with older maternal age. It is characterized by craniofacial abnormalities including micrognathia, a narrow bifrontal diameter, low-set ears and a small mouth, clenched hands with the fifth finger overlapping the fourth, talipes causing 'rocker bottom' feet and weakness. Most cases die in utero and are spontaneously aborted. Tetralogy of Fallot is sometimes seen. Holoprosencephaly is a feature of Patau's syndrome.

A 3. **A.** false **B.** false **C.** false **D.** false **E.** true

Cri du chat syndrome is due to partial deletion of the short arm of chromosome 5 (5p-syndrome). The infants are of low birth weight with a cry like a cat. All have low intelligence and microcephaly.

A 4. **A.** false **B.** true **C.** false **D.** true **E.** false

Mosaicism accounts for only about 1% of Trisomy 21 (Down's syndrome) cases. Robertsonian translocation accounts for less than 5% of cases, the vast majority being due to non-disjunction. If the father is a translocation carrier, the recurrence risk is 2.5%.

A 5. **A.** true **B.** false **C.** false **D.** false **E.** true

Cystic fibrosis is the result of a three-base pair deletion, and Duchenne muscular dystrophy an increase in the normal tandem repeats. Sickle cell anaemia is a missense mutation involving a substitution of valine for glutamic acid at position 6 of the beta-globin polypeptide chain.

A 6.   **A.** false   **B.** true   **C.** false   **D.** false   **E.** true

The upper part of the motor nucleus of the facial nerve controls the lower facial muscles, and receives contralateral fibres only, hence unilateral lesions of the motor cortex affect the lower part of the contralateral face. The upper face would not be affected by such lesions as the lower part of the motor nucleus of the facial nerve (which controls the upper facial muscles), receives both crossed and uncrossed fibres. The chorda tympani branch of the facial nerve transmits taste from the anterior two-thirds of the tongue. The facial nerve conveys secretomotor fibres to the submandibular and sublingual salivary glands and the lacrimal gland.

Anatomy for Anaesthetists. Ed. Ellis H & Feldman S, 6th edn 1993, Oxford: Blackwell Science, pp. 281–6.

A 7.   **A.** false   **B.** false   **C.** true   **D.** true   **E.** true

The occulomotor (IIIrd) cranial nerve supplies all the extrinsic eye muscles except lateral rectus and superior oblique, and conveys the preganglionic parasympathetic fibres for the pupil sphincter and the ciliary muscle. Complete division of the nerve will thus cause a divergent squint due to the unopposed action of the superior oblique and lateral rectus muscles.

Anatomy for Anaesthetists. Ed. Ellis H & Feldman S, 6th edn 1993, Oxford: Blackwell Science, pp. 256–8.

A 8.   **A.** false   **B.** true   **C.** true   **D.** false   **E.** true

Meningomyelocele is a protrusion of both meninges and nerves through a vertebral defect. Other associated problems are bladder and bowel dysfunction, lower limb paralysis, scoliosis and hip dislocation.

A 9.   **A.** true   **B.** true   **C.** true   **D.** true   **E.** true

A **10.** **A.** true **B.** true **C.** false **D.** false **E.** true

In childhood absence epilepsy there is a positive family history in around 40% of cases. The usual age affected is from 3 to 10 years, and it is more common in girls.

A **11.** **A.** false **B.** true **C.** true **D.** false **E.** true

Sodium valproate is first-line therapy in generalized tonic-clonic seizures and atypical absences. Side-effects include hyperphagia (causing weight gain), thrombocytopenia and tremor (both dose-dependent) and frequently causes a transient elevation of liver enzymes but can occasionally result in fulminant hepatic failure.

A **12.** **A.** false **B.** false **C.** false **D.** false **E.** false

The forward parachute and lateral propping reflex both remain present for life. The palmar grasp disappears at 3–4 months, the stepping reflex at 2 months and the Moro reflex at 4–5 months.

A **13.** **A.** true **B.** true **C.** true **D.** false **E.** false

Dermoids usually straddle the corneo-scleral limbus and may be associated with Goldenhar's syndrome. Congenital hereditary endothelial dystrophy is an uncommon hereditary dystrophy, with an onset at birth with corneal clouding and oedema.

A **14.** **A.** false **B.** true **C.** true **D.** true **E.** true

Galactosaemia can cause leucocoria via cataract formation. Buphthalmos causes corneal clouding due to corneal oedema.

A **15.** **A.** false **B.** true **C.** true **D.** true **E.** false

Fetal haemoglobin is composed of HbF and HbA2. HbF contains α 2–γ 2 polypeptide chains.

A **16.** **A.** true **B.** true **C.** false **D.** false **E.** true

Diseases affecting ileal absorption can cause B12 deficiency. These include Crohn's disease and intestinal TB. Trimethoprim and phenytoin are both anti-folate drugs and therefore cause a folate deficiency. Fish tapeworm absorbs the B12.

A **17.** **A.** true **B.** true **C.** false **D.** true **E.** true

Hereditary spherocytosis is caused by abnormalities of the red cell membrane skeletal proteins. There are multiple known defects, which result in varying degrees of haemolysis and therefore it may present with neonatal jaundice if haemolysis is high or later during childhood or even adulthood if the disease is milder. Due to the haemolysis, the reticulocyte count is raised to about 5–20%.

A **18.** **A.** true **B.** true **C.** true **D.** false **E.** false

A high platelet count is seen post-splenectomy. In addition, a lymphocytosis, irregular contracted red cells and Howell-Jolly bodies are seen.

A **19.** **A.** false **B.** false **C.** false **D.** true **E.** false

A **20.** **A.** false **B.** false **C.** false **D.** true **E.** false

Polymorphonuclear granulocytes make up about 70% of the total normal blood leucocytes, and over 95% of them are neutrophils. They live only 2–3 days, and are involved in non-specific immunity, predominantly employing phagocytosis of micro-organisms and debris.

A **21.** **A.** false **B.** true **C.** false **D.** true **E.** true

Urticaria pigmentosa is one of the most common forms of cutaneous mastocytosis, a disorder involving proliferation of mast cells. No treatment is usually required and the disorder generally resolves spontaneously over a number of years. Systemic symptoms due to histamine release may occur.

A **22.** **A.** true **B.** true **C.** false **D.** true **E.** false

Phenylketonuria is due to low or absent phenylalanine hydroxylase, resulting in an accumulation of phenylalanine. It is managed with a low phenylalanine diet (some phenylalanine must be given as it is not synthesized in the body). Classically, there is a musty smell. Strict adherence to the diet during pregnancy is important to prevent damage to the fetus.

A 23. **A.** true   **B.** false   **C.** true   **D.** true   **E.** true

Homocystinuria is due to a deficiency of the enzyme cystathione synthase, and results in an accumulation of homocysteine and methionine. It is a disorder of amino acid metabolism. It causes mental retardation, a Marfanoid habitus, arterial and venous thromboembolism, and downwards lens subluxation.

A 24. **A.** true   **B.** true   **C.** false   **D.** false   **E.** false

Wilson's disease is a disorder of copper transport and is inherited in autosomal recessive fashion. Relatives can and should be screened as they may have mild clinical features and require treatment.

A 25. **A.** false   **B.** true   **C.** false   **D.** true   **E.** false

Red cell aplasia occurs in Blackfan-Diamond syndrome. Metaphyseal not epiphyseal dysostosis occurs. Average life expectancy is about 35 years and treatment with GCSF or stem cell transplant may increase this.

A 26. **A.** false   **B.** true   **C.** true   **D.** true   **E.** false

Bleeding is almost universally painless when occurring with a polyp. CHRPE (congenital hypertrophy of the retinal pigment epithelium) is an association with the APC (adenomatous polyposis coli) gene in 58–75% of cases and may be used in risk assessment. Peutz-Jegher's syndrome does not lead to GI tumours but does lead to malignant tumours outside the GI tract in up to 50% of cases. Pseudopolyps and inflammatory polyps in the healing phase of UC (ulcerative colitis) are well recognized.

A 27. **A.** true   **B.** false   **C.** false   **D.** true   **E.** false

Oral ulceration is present in 90% of those with Behçet's disease. Recurrent aphthous ulceration is mainly of idiopathic aetiology.

Perioral and perianal lesions occur in acrodermatitis enteropathica associated with a low zinc level.

Rule D, Speight P. Chapter 24. In *Pediatric Gastrointestinal Disease*. Ed. Walker A *et al*. St Louis: Mosby, 1996.

A 28. A. true   **B.** false   **C.** true   **D.** true   **E.** false

Even if small amounts of urobilinogen are seen in the urine (usually with unconjugated hyperbilirubinaemia), in biliary atresia this is not usually manifest until after the first day of life. The Kasai procedure is effective whether the biliary atresia is intra- or extra-hepatic.

Roberts E. Chapter 2. In *Disorders of the Liver and Biliary System in Childhood*. Ed. Kelly D. Oxford: Blackwell Science, 1999.

A 29. A. true   **B.** false   **C.** true   **D.** false   **E.** true

After administration of penicillamine, the 24-hour urinary copper excretion, which is already raised, increases even more. Serum caeruloplasmin is raised and serum copper can be raised or normal. Liver biopsy characteristically reveals marked periportal copper deposition, and more recently, the gene has been mapped to chromosome 13q14–21. As it is autosomal dominant, other family members should be screened. The underlying mechanism appears to be a defect of hepatocyte transport of copper into the caeruloplasmin compartment. HLA-A3 is found in association with 72% of haemochromatosis – HLA-B7 in Australia and HLA-B14 in France are also seen.

Tanner S. Chapter 10. In *Disorders of the Liver and Biliary System in Childhood*. Ed. Kelly D. Oxford: Blackwell Science, 1999.

A 30. A. false   **B.** true   **C.** true   **D.** false   **E.** false

The cardiac axis is right and anterior in the neonate. Children are unable to alter stroke volume very much and therefore rely on the heart rate to alter blood flow. Causes of a fourth heart sound include long-standing hypertension and ischaemic heart disease.

A. true   **B.** false   **C.** false   **D.** false   **E.** true

The causes of a right-sided aortic arch are: Fallot's tetralogy, truncus arteriosus, pulmonary atresia with a ventricular septal defect, congenital vascular ring and 22q11 deletion.

A 32.   **A.** false   **B.** false   **C.** true   **D.** false   **E.** false

Pulmonary artery band, coarctation of the aorta repair and patent ductus arteriosus ligation all result in a left thoracotomy scar.

A 33.   **A.** false   **B.** true   **C.** false   **D.** true   **E.** false

Pulmonary atresia with an intact ventricular septum is always duct-dependent and therefore requires emergency treatment with prostaglandin E2 in the neonate. If there is a ventricular septal defect, blood is able to mix via this. The chest X-ray shows a right-sided aortic arch and a 'coeur en sabot' finding.

A 34.   **A.** false   **B.** true   **C.** true   **D.** true   **E.** true

Tetralogy of Fallot may present within the first few days of life with cyanosis, or later with detection of a murmur or with hypercyanotic spells. There is an ejection systolic murmur at the upper left sternal edge. Corrective surgery is performed between 4 months and 1 year.

A 35.   **A.** true   **B.** false   **C.** false   **D.** false   **E.** false

Fructose, glucose, galactose and amino acids are reabsorbed in the proximal renal tubule.

A 36.   **A.** true   **B.** true   **C.** false   **D.** true   **E.** false

In distal renal tubular acidosis, there is a failure of excretion of H^+ by the distal renal tubule. There is hypocalcaemia, with hypercalciuria and high serum chloride. Osteomalacia is seen but not clinical rickets. Nephrocalcinosis and renal stones occur.

A 37.   **A.** false   **B.** false   **C.** false   **D.** false   **E.** false

Nephrotic syndrome is more common in boys. The urine albumin: creatinine ratio is >200 mg/mmol. Frothy urine, however, is rare.

Exam 3

Answers

In minimal change nephrotic syndrome, C3 is normal and there are no red cell casts.

A 38. A. false **B.** false **C.** false **D.** true **E.** true

Fanconi's syndrome is a generalized defect in proximal renal tubular function. There is a hyperchloraemic, hypokalaemic metabolic acidosis. There is increased urine loss of bicarbonate, phosphate, sodium, calcium, potassium, urate, glucose and amino acids.

A 39. A. true **B.** true **C.** false **D.** true **E.** true

In a child, the lungs have less elastin and are less compliant, making airway collapse more probable. The alveoli are smaller and fewer in number. The rib cage is more pliable (and the ribs more horizontal), making it less efficient for ventilation. The airways are smaller with greater resistance, increasing the work of breathing and susceptibility to airway disease.

A 40. A. false **B.** false **C.** true **D.** false **E.** false

In acute laryngo-tracheo-bronchitis (croup) adrenaline causes a rapid improvement but can be followed by a rebound increased stridor in 30–45 minutes. Croup is most common in 1- to 2-year-olds. Arterial blood gas measurement is an invasive distressing procedure, which would make the symptoms worse and should be avoided. Assessment should include checking for signs of hypoxia, drowsiness or rapid clinical deterioration (features of severity and indications for possible intubation and ventilation).

A 41. A. false **B.** false **C.** true **D.** true **E.** false

Anti-nRNP may be positive. It is positive in 100% of cases in mixed connective tissue disease. Decreased C3 is a sign of active disease. Gottron's papules are a feature of dermatomyositis.

A 42. A. true **B.** true **C.** true **D.** false **E.** false

Associated anomalies occur with congenital diaphragmatic hernia in up to 30% of cases. These include central nervous system anomalies, oesophageal atresia, omphalocele, cardiovascular lesions and certain syndromes including Trisomy 13, 18 and 21, Brachmann-de Lange syndrome and Fryn syndrome.

A. false **B.** false **C.** true **D.** true **E.** true

In first-order kinetics, a constant proportion of drug is metabolized in a given time period. The absolute amount eliminated is greatest when plasma concentration is greatest and the rate of elimination and elimination half-life are constant, irrespective of plasma concentration.

A 44. **A.** false **B.** true **C.** false **D.** true **E.** true

Tacrolimus is a calcineurin inhibitor. It is both more nephrotoxic and more neurotoxic than ciclosporin.

A 45. **A.** false **B.** false **C.** true **D.** false **E.** true

Desferioxamine is given subcutaneously. Iron excretion is enhanced by administration of vitamin C. It can cause hypotension (especially if given too rapidly by intravenous injection).

A 46. **A.** false **B.** false **C.** false **D.** true **E.** false

An organic cause is only found in around 10% of cases. Siblings have a 2–3% prevalence of autism, and monozygotic twins have 60% concordance. Developmental stasis or regression is seen in 25–30% at 15–18 months of age.

A 47. **A.** false **B.** false **C.** true **D.** true **E.** true

Hydrops fetalis may be caused by intrauterine infection with cytomegalovirus, toxoplasmosis, syphilis, parvovirus B19, leptospirosis and Chagas disease.
Other causes of hydrops fetalis are haematological (Rhesus and other incompatability), cardiovascular (e.g. SVT, heart failure), pulmonary (e.g. CAM lung), neonatal tumour (e.g. congenital neuroblastoma), hepatic (e.g. hepatitis), renal (e.g. posterior urethral valves), gastrointestinal (e.g. atresias, volvulus), metabolic (e.g. maternal diabetes mellitus) and malformations (e.g. Turner syndrome, Trisomy 18).

A 48. **A.** false **B.** false **C.** false **D.** true **E.** false

The risk of fetal infection with toxoplasmosis is inversely related to gestational age, the highest risk being 65% during the third

Exam 3

Answers

trimester. The severity of fetal infection is also related to gestational age, with the highest risk at 24–30 weeks' gestation. Infection particularly affects the developing brain, causing diffusely scattered intracranial calcification and neurological consequences including developmental delay, microcephaly, hydrocephalus and seizures.

A **49.** **A.** false **B.** false **C.** true **D.** true **E.** true

Approximately 30% of women have vaginal colonization with Group B β-haemolytic streptococci. Only 1% of infants colonized during delivery develop sepsis, however. Colonized infants born to mothers with premature rupture of membranes or with pyrexia are at greater risk of sepsis if inadequate labour prophylaxis is given.

A **50.** **A.** true **B.** true **C.** true **D.** true **E.** false

Infants with intrauterine growth retardation are at greater risk of perinatal asphyxia, hypoglycaemia, hypothermia, infection, hypocalcaemia and polycythaemia. Studies have shown a long-term increase in behavioural and learning difficulties.

Strauss RS. Adult functional outcome of those born small for gestational age: Twenty-six year follow-up of the 1970 British Birth Cohort. *JAMA* 2000; **283**: 625–32.

A **51.** **A.** false **B.** true **C.** false **D.** false **E.** false

Colostrum is lower in total fat composition and lactose than mature human breast milk. It is higher in phospholipids, cholesterol and protein concentration. It is very rich in immunoglobulins, particularly secretory IgA.

A **52.** **A.** false **B.** true **C.** false **D.** false **E.** false

The adrenal medulla secretes adrenaline and noradrenaline. The adrenal cortex secretes the mineralocorticoids, glucocorticoids and anabolic and sex hormones.

A **53.** **A.** false **B.** true **C.** true **D.** false **E.** true

Features of diabetes insipidus include lots of wet nappies, dehydration, rapid weight loss, failure to thrive and collapse in infants. There may be a history of intermittent fevers. In older children, polydipsia, polyuria, new onset nocturia, lack of perspiration, anorexia and dehydration are seen. Glycosuria would be suggestive of diabetes mellitus.

A 54. **A.** true **B.** false **C.** false **D.** false **E.** false

Multiple endocrine neoplasia (MEN) type I is characterized by pancreatic islet cell adenomas (producing insulin and gastrin), prolactinomas and parathyroid adenomas. Phaeochromocytoma and medullary thyroid carcinoma are seen in MEN II, and multiple mucosal neuromas in addition to the features of MEN II in MEN III.

A 55. **A.** false **B.** false **C.** true **D.** false **E.** true

In girls, puberty onset is usually between 8 and 13 years. The first sign in girls is breast development (thelarche) and in boys, testicular enlargement. In girls, menstruation usually commences at breast stage 4, on average at 12.2 years of age.

A 56. **A.** true **B.** false **C.** false **D.** true **E.** true

McCune-Albright syndrome is a syndrome of endocrine dysfunction due to a mutation in the gene encoding a subunit of Gs (the G protein that stimulates cAMP formation) causing stimulation of endocrine receptors (e.g. ACTH, TSH, LH and FSH receptors). The clinical features are variable and include multiple endocrine anomalies including precocious puberty, hyperthyroidism and Cushing's syndrome. There may also be café-au-lait lesions (large, irregular and often to the midline), osteomalacia, and hepatic involvement.

A 57. **A.** false **B.** false **C.** false **D.** false **E.** false

Tetanus vaccine is a toxoid. It can be given to immunocompromised children. Once the primary course has been given, a booster is given after 3 years and a further booster after 10 years. This gives protection for life unless there is a high-risk injury.

A 58. **A.** false **B.** false **C.** true **D.** true **E.** false

Syphilis infection during pregnancy has a transmission of nearly 100%. The Jarisch-Herxheimer reaction is an acute systemic reaction when syphilis is treated and it can occur in congenital syphilis cases. Blindness can result from a keratitis followed by corneal opacification. There is a thrombocytopenia.

A 59. **A.** true **B.** true **C.** false **D.** true **E.** false

Scarlet fever is caused by Group A streptococcal infection (*Streptococcus pyogenes*), and is due to exotoxin production. Classically, there is sudden onset of high fever, vomiting, pharyngitis, headache and toxicity. The tonsils are red and may develop an exudate. The tongue is initially white (white strawberry tongue), and after several days desquamates and becomes red (red strawberry tongue). The scarlatiniform rash appears initially on the neck, groin and axillae and rapidly generalizes. Abdominal pain may be present and if this precedes the rash, confusion with a surgical condition can occur.

A 60. **A.** true **B.** false **C.** false **D.** true **E.** true

Up to 75% of affected individuals produce cold agglutinins. The chest X-ray often looks unexpectedly severe.

Q 1. **The following are true of Down's syndrome**

A. Brushfield spots are pathognomonic
B. The average IQ is 70
C. They have an increased incidence of atherosclerotic heart disease
D. Some develop dementia secondary to amyloid deposition
E. The saggital cranial suture is separated

Q 2. **The following are true**

A. The likelihood that a newborn infant with a single transverse palmar crease has Down's syndrome is 1 in 60
B. Neurofibromatosis has the highest known mutation rate per gamete
C. Mitochondrial DNA abnormalities are passed on only via the father
D. In a Robertsonian translocation Down's syndrome the chance of recurrence is 50% if the father is a translocation carrier
E. Expression of mitochondrial DNA disorders is variable

Q 3. **The following conditions are associated with advanced paternal age**

A. Achondroplasia
B. Cystic fibrosis
C. Apert sydrome
D. Marfan syndrome
E. Beckwith-Wiedemann syndrome

Q 4. **The following conditions are causes of a macrosomic infant**

A. Beckwith-Wiedemann syndrome
B. Weaver syndrome
C. Baller-Gerold syndrome
D. Prader-Willi syndrome
E. Bardet-Biedl syndrome

Q 5. **The following developmental terms are correctly defined**

A. A malformation is a single prior anomaly or mechanical factor causing a pattern of abnormalities

B. A disruption is a primary defect involving abnormal cellular organization or function

C. Dysplasia is an abnormality due to mechanical forces

D. Deformation is a primary defect resulting from intrinsic abnormal development

E. A sequence is a destructive process of a previously normal structure

Q 6. **The following conditions cause an elevated CSF protein**

A. Peripheral neuropathy

B. Krabbe disease

C. Lead poisoning

D. Encephalitis

E. Post-infectious encephalopathy

Q 7. **The following are associated with cerebral palsy**

A. Good 5-minute Apgar score (7–10) in 25% of patients

B. Nystagmus

C. Attention deficit disorder

D. Easily startled in infancy

E. Poor 20-minute Apgar score (0–3) in 60% of patients

Q 8. **The histopathology of the lesions in adenoma sebaceum shows them to be**

A. Fibroadenomas

B. Angiofibromas

C. Dermatofibromas

D. Angiosarcomas

E. Angiolipomas

Q 9. **In tuberous sclerosis**

A. Angiofibromas develop from age 10 years

B. Less than a quarter have café-au-lait macules at birth

C. 80% develop periungual fibromas during teenage years

D. By age 5 years around one-third will have a Shagreen patch

E. Around 50% have seizures

Q 10. Absence seizures

A. Have a short post-ictal phase
B. Require no treatment
C. May involve eyelid fluttering
D. Are seen in 10% of children
E. Have a typical 1 per second spike and wave EEG

Q 11. The following are true of cerebral palsy

A. Most infants with cerebral palsy have identifiable risk factors
B. Most cases of cerebral palsy are related to delivery
C. Severe colic is common in infants with cerebral palsy
D. Mental retardation is present in one-third of affected infants
E. Seizures are present in one-third of affected infants

Q 12. The following shapes can be drawn by the specified ages in a normally developing child

A. Square – 3.5 yrs
B. Triangle – 4 years
C. Diamond – 6 years
D. 4-dimensional rectangle – 9 years
E. Circle – 3 years

Q 13. Regarding retinoblastoma

A. The incidence is 1 in 30 000 live births
B. 40% are sporadic
C. The retinoblastoma (*RB1*) gene is on chromosome 15
D. Overall survival is 75%
E. In the hereditary form there is incomplete penetrance

Q 14. Regarding optic atrophy in children

A. A pale disc with attenuated vasculature is seen on fundoscopy
B. The pupillary light reflex is normal
C. It can be caused by leukaemia
D. There may be defective colour vision
E. Is a feature of DIDMOAD syndrome

Q 15. **The following are causes of a low erythrocyte sedimentation ratio (ESR)**

A. Cardiac failure
B. Sickle cell anaemia
C. Nephrotic syndrome
D. Liver disease
E. Cyanotic congenital heart failure

Q 16. **Howell-Jolly bodies are seen in**

A. Iron deficiency anaemia
B. Pyruvate kinase deficiency
C. Microangiopathic anaemia
D. Abetalipoproteinaemia
E. Sideroblastic anaemia

Q 17. **Regarding von Willebrand's disease**

A. Bleeding time may be normal
B. Symptoms can be affected by stress
C. Ristocetin-induced platelet aggregation is reduced
D. Factor VIIIc activity is normal
E. Inheritance is autosomal recessive

Q 18. **The following conditions can cause a reduced factor V level**

A. DIC
B. Vitamin K deficiency
C. Liver disease
D. Haemophilia B
E. Haemophilia C

Q 19. **Haemophilia C**

A. Is due to factor VI deficiency
B. Is of X-linked recessive inheritance
C. Is most common in Afro-Caribbeans
D. Is a cause of post-operative haemorrhage
E. Can present with epistaxis

Q 20. **The clinical features of hyper-IgE syndrome include**

A. Low C4
B. Osteopenia

C. Thrombocytopenia

D. Recurrent boils

E. Prolonged retention of primary teeth

Q 21. The following conditions can cause neonatal vesicles

A. Benign cephalic histiocytosis

B. Keratosis pilaris

C. Urticaria pigmentosum

D. Erythema toxicum neonatorum

E. Incontinentia pigmentii

Q 22. Alkaptonuria is characterized by

A. Pale stools

B. Cataracts

C. Convulsions

D. Elevated urine methionine levels

E. Ochronosis

Q 23. Cystinosis is characterized by

A. Hypertension

B. Blue urine

C. Rickets

D. Cataracts

E. Renal stones

Q 24. Glycogen storage diseases

A. Are a cause of osteoporosis

B. Are managed with a low protein diet

C. Present with hypoglycaemia during intercurrent illness

D. Are a cause of hepatomegaly

E. Include Pompe disease

Q 25. The following are true about gastric acid production

A. Sympathomimetics increase gastric acid production

B. Secretin inhibits gastric acid production

C. *Helicobacter pylori* colonization of the gastric lining increases gastric acid production

D. Vagal nerve stimulation increases the pH of the intragastric milieu

E. Pancreatic β-cells increase the pH of the intragastric milieu

Q 26. In an infant with intestinal lymphangiectasia

A. A small bowel biopsy will reveal minimal or no lacteals
B. The cause may be constrictive pericarditis
C. An association is Klippel-Trenauney-Weber syndrome
D. Faecal α-1-antitrypsin may be decreased
E. Mental retardation and regression are common

Q 27. Chronic pancreatitis in children

A. Occurs in ascariasis
B. Occurs in Wilson's disease
C. Will display Cullen's sign if prolonged
D. Is predisposed to by cystinosis
E. Is predisposed to by cystinuria

Q 28. Recognized poor prognostic factors in children presenting with fulminant liver failure include

A. Age under 10 years
B. Paracetamol-induced liver failure
C. Marked hepatomegaly with evidence of portal hypertension
D. Urine output of less than 0.3 mL/kg/hour
E. Parents who are consanguineous

Q 29. Treatment of potential or actual variceal bleeding in childhood can involve the following

A. Transjugular intrahepatic porto-systemic shunt
B. Endoscopic variceal band ligation
C. With a Sengstaken-Blakemore tube, use of the balloon only
D. Neomycin for gut sterilization to aid in the prevention of hepatic encephalopathy
E. Intravenous octreotide infusion

Q 30. An ejection click may be due to

A. Truncus arteriosus
B. Tetralogy of Fallot
C. Tricuspid atresia
D. Pulmonary stenosis
E. Aortic stenosis

Q 31. In a dilated cardiomyopathy

    A. An increased ejection fraction is seen on echocardiogram
    B. Left ventricular hypertrophy is seen on the ECG
    C. Anticoagulation is not indicated
    D. The right ventricle is not affected
    E. Friedreich's ataxia is a cause

Q 32. In the neonatal period, prostaglandin E2 is contraindicated for

    A. Critical pulmonary stenosis
    B. Total anomalous pulmonary venous drainage
    C. Hypoplastic left heart syndrome
    D. Interrupted aortic arch
    E. Tricuspid atresia with intact ventricular septum

Q 33. A single second heart sound may be present in

    A. Pulmonary stenosis
    B. Mitral regurgitation
    C. Atrial septal defect
    D. Normal newborns
    E. Aortic stenosis

Q 34. The following are features of Ebstein's anomaly

    A. Proximally placed tricuspid valve
    B. Ventricular septal defect
    C. Wolf-Parkinson-White syndrome type A
    D. Abnormal mitral valve
    E. Extrasystoles

Q 35. Regarding the development of the renal tract

    A. The pronephros is non-functional in the human embryo
    B. The urogenital ridges develop during the fourth week of development
    C. The mesonephros produces dilute urine
    D. The ureteric bud gives rise to the Bowman's capsules
    E. The nephrogenic cap develops into the ureters

Q 36. In Henoch-Schönlein purpura

    A. The joints of hands and feet are classically affected
    B. Melaena is present in at least 50% of cases

C. Thrombocytopenia is common

D. Nearly 50% of the intussusceptions are ileo-ileal

E. Epididymitis is seen in approximately one-third of males

Q 37. In congenital horseshoe kidney

A. The upper poles are usually united

B. Ureteric obstruction is present in up to one-third of cases

C. The ureters pass posterior to the bridge

D. It is seen in 1 in 1000 people

E. It is associated with Turner syndrome

Q 38. In post-streptococcal glomerulonephritis

A. It is seen during streptococcal upper respiratory tract infections

B. Microscopic haematuria usually continues for up to 1 year

C. Renal biopsy should be done

D. Severe hypertension is usually present

E. It should be treated with oral penicillin

Q 39. In the development of the respiratory tract

A. The cartilaginous tracheal rings develop from the splanchnopleuric mesenchyme during the eighth week of gestation

B. The lung buds develop in the sixth week of gestation

C. Type II pneumocytes appear in the fifth month of gestation

D. The trachea and oesophagus separate in the third week of gestation

E. New pulmonary lobules continue to form postnatally until puberty

Q 40. Lung surfactant

A. Increases surface tension at low lung volumes

B. Acts to prevents atelectasis

C. Is composed of glycoproteins

D. Is manufactured by type I pneumocytes

E. Equalizes pressure in connected alveoli

Q 41. In rheumatic fever

    A. A prolonged PR interval is one of the minor diagnostic criteria

    B. The arthritis is painless

    C. The severity of the carditis is often inversely proportional to the severity of the arthritis

    D. The arthritis usually resolves within 4 weeks

    E. Erythema marginatum is seen in 10% of cases

Q 42. Malrotation

    A. Develops during the second month of gestation

    B. May present as a protein-losing enteropathy

    C. Is asymptomatic to adolescence in up to 50% of cases

    D. Is not treated unless symptomatic

    E. Is caused by incomplete rotation of the intestine around the inferior mesenteric artery

Q 43. Lamotrigine

    A. Causes photosensitivity

    B. If given, liver function should be monitored

    C. Is used to treat partial seizures

    D. May cause influenza-like symptoms

    E. Is effective in gastro-oesophageal reflux

Q 44. Penicillamine is used to treat

    A. Cystinuria

    B. Lead poisoning

    C. Dermatomyositis

    D. Nephrotic syndrome

    E. Haemolytic anaemia

Q 45. The following are characteristic of zero-order kinetics

    A. They occur when the enzyme responsible for the reaction is saturated

    B. A constant amount of drug is metabolized in a given period of time

    C. The reaction is represented by a linear relationship

D. The rate of elimination is independent of the plasma concentration

E. The absolute amount eliminated is the same regardless of plasma concentration

Q 46. The following features are seen in Asperger's syndrome

A. Clumsiness in infancy
B. Good non-verbal communication skills
C. Late walking
D. Language delay
E. Literal interpretation of conversations

Q 47. Respiratory physiology in the neonate, compared with the adult shows

A. A decreased ventilatory response to hypercarbia
B. 2–3 times greater oxygen consumption
C. Higher physiological dead space
D. Lower airway resistance
E. Lower lung compliance

Q 48. Congenital lobar emphysema

A. May not present until age 5 months
B. Responds to treatment with surfactant
C. Usually affects the lower lobes
D. Is associated with CHD
E. May be familial

Q 49. Nitric oxide

A. Is normally produced in the endothelial cells
B. Is produced during the conversion of arginine and oxygen to citrulline
C. Activates guanyl cyclase
D. Causes pulmonary arteriolar smooth muscle contraction
E. Is inactivated to methaemoglobin

Q 50. The following conditions are associated with increased maternal serum alpha-fetoprotein

A. Intrauterine growth retardation
B. Renal agenesis

C. Cystic hygroma

D. Trisomy 18

E. Turner syndrome

Q 51. The following amino acids are essential for the preterm infant

A. Leucine

B. Methionine

C. Tryptophan

D. Linoleic acid

E. Linolenic acid

Q 52. Recognized features of type 1 diabetes mellitus include

A. 30% identical twin concordance

B. A 1 in 40 risk of a sibling developing the disease

C. A risk of 1 in 30 for the child of a mother with type 1 diabetes

D. A prevalence of 1 in 1000 in the UK

E. The presence of circulating islet cell antibodies

Q 53. Causes of the syndrome of inappropriate antidiuretic hormone secretion (SIADH) include

A. Cystic fibrosis

B. Craniopharyngioma

C. Morphine

D. Lithium

E. Demeclocycline

Q 54. Features of autoimmune polyendocrine syndrome type II include

A. Adrenal insufficiency

B. Diabetes mellitus

C. Chronic lymphocytic thyroiditis

D. Hypoparathyroidism

E. Mucocutaneous candidiasis

Q 55. The following are causes of primary amenorrhoea without secondary sexual characteristics

A. Turner syndrome

B. Gonadal dysgenesis

C. Empty sella syndrome
D. Testicular feminization syndrome
E. Hypothyroidism

Q 56. Regarding delayed puberty

A. It is defined in girls as failure of onset of any signs of puberty by age 14 years
B. It may be caused by malnutrition
C. It may be caused by congenital adrenal hyperplasia due to 11-hydroxylase deficiency
D. It may be caused by hypothyroidism
E. It is most common in girls

Q 57. The following are contraindications to pertussis vaccination

A. Epilepsy
B. Surgical procedure within the previous 4 weeks
C. Family history of adverse reaction to pertussis vaccine
D. Current treatment with amoxicillin
E. Haemodialysis for renal failure

Q 58. Regarding diphtheria

A. *Corynebacterium diphtheriae* mitis type causes the most severe disease
B. The toxin subunit B produces the clinical disease
C. The incubation period is 2 weeks
D. May result in a fatal myocarditis
E. Carriage of organisms in healthy individuals does not occur

Q 59. Otitis media

A. Is usually viral
B. Is not associated with a residual middle ear effusion at 2 weeks in most children
C. Usually causes temporary deafness
D. If bacterial is often due to *Moxarella catarrhalis*
E. May be complicated by facial nerve paralysis

Lymphadenitis in an otherwise healthy child

A. Does not need to be investigated
B. Is most commonly due to TB infection
C. If erythematous and tender in the cervical area is suggestive of mycobacterium infection
D. If swollen and tender in the cervical area suggests cat scratch disease
E. If fluctuant suggests an abscess

A 1. **A.** false **B.** false **C.** false **D.** true **E.** true

Brushfield spots are only present in three-quarters of Down's syndrome children, and are also found in 7–10% of newborn Caucasians. The average IQ is 54 (35–65). They have a reduced incidence of atherosclerotic heart disease.

A 2. **A.** true **B.** true **C.** false **D.** false **E.** true

Mitochondrial DNA abnormalities are passed on only via the mother because the mitochondria are in the cytoplasm of the egg but not the sperm. The expression of these disorders is variable because mosaicism is common. In a Robertsonian translocation Down's syndrome the chance of recurrence is 100% if the father is a translocation carrier.

A 3. **A.** true **B.** false **C.** true **D.** true **E.** false

Achondroplasia, Apert syndrome and Marfan syndrome are all associated with advanced paternal age.

A 4. **A.** true **B.** true **C.** false **D.** true **E.** true

Infants of diabetic mothers are also macrosomic.

A 5. **A.** false **B.** false **C.** false **D.** false **E.** false

A malformation is a primary defect resulting from intrinsic abnormal development. A disruption is a destructive process of a previously normal structure. Dysplasia is a primary defect involving abnormal cellular organization or function. Deformation is an abnormality due to mechanical forces. A sequence is a single prior anomaly or mechanical factor causing a pattern of abnormalities.

A 6. **A.** true **B.** true **C.** true **D.** true **E.** true

Other common causes of raised CSF protein are acute bacterial meningitis, TB meningitis, multiple sclerosis, Guillain-Barré syndrome, stroke and uraemia.

A 7. **A.** false **B.** true **C.** true **D.** true **E.** true

A good 5-minute Apgar score (7–10) was seen in nearly 75% of patients with cerebral palsy.

Nelson KB, Ellenberg JH. Apgar scores as predictors of chronic neurological disability. *Pediatrics* 1981; **68**: 36–44.

A 8. **A.** true **B.** false **C.** false **D.** false **E.** false

A 9. **A.** false **B.** true **C.** false **D.** true **E.** false

Angiofibromas develop from age 2 to 5 years. Periungual fibromas develop during the teenage years in up to 50%. Over 80% have seizures, most commonly infantile spasms.

A 10. **A.** false **B.** false **C.** true **D.** false **E.** false

Absence seizures have no post-ictal phase. They may require anti-epileptic medication. The EEG shows a 3 per second spike and wave pattern.

A 11. **A.** false **B.** false **C.** true **D.** false **E.** true

Few cases of cerebral palsy are related to delivery and most have no identifiable risk factors. Severe colic is seen in around one-third of infants with cerebral palsy. Mental retardation is present in two-thirds of affected infants.

A 12. **A.** false **B.** false **C.** false **D.** false **E.** true

A normal child can draw a square by 4.5 years, a triangle by 5 years, a diamond by 7 years and a 4-dimensional rectangle by 12 years.

A 13. **A.** false **B.** false **C.** false **D.** false **E.** true

The incidence of retinoblastoma is 1 in 16 000 live births. 60% are sporadic. The retinoblastoma (*RB1*) gene is on chromosome 13q. Overall survival is above 90%.

A **14.** **A.** true   **B.** false   **C.** true   **D.** true   **E.** true

It may be associated with an abnormal pupillary light reflex if severe.

A **15.** **A.** true   **B.** true   **C.** true   **D.** true   **E.** true

A low ESR can be the result of reduced concentration of large proteins as in liver disease, nephrotic syndrome and cardiac failure, an abnormal red cell membrane as in sickle cell anaemia or in polycythaemia as occurs in congenital cyanotic heart disease.

A **16.** **A.** false   **B.** true   **C.** true   **D.** true   **E.** true

Howell-Jolly bodies are seen in hyposplenism and post splenectomy.

A **17.** **A.** true   **B.** true   **C.** true   **D.** false   **E.** false

Von Willebrand's disease is a heterogeneous group of disorders involving the von Willebrand factor (vWF). It is of autosomal dominant inheritance with variable expression. Factor VIIIc activity is reduced. In mild disease the bleeding time may be normal, though it is prolonged in more severe disease.

A **18.** **A.** true   **B.** false   **C.** true   **D.** false   **E.** false

Factor V is produced by the liver, and therefore liver disease will cause reduced levels. The vitamin K-dependent factors are factors II, VII, IX and X and do not include factor V.

A **19.** **A.** false   **B.** false   **C.** false   **D.** true   **E.** true

Haemophilia C is factor XI deficiency. It is transmitted as an incomplete autosomal recessive disease, and only homozygotes are clinically affected. It is most commonly seen in Ashkenazi Jews. It presents with epistaxis, haematuria and menorrhagia, and with post-operative bleeding. Spontaneous bleeds are rare.

A **20.** **A.** false   **B.** true   **C.** false   **D.** true   **E.** true

The hyper-IgE syndrome features recurrent sinopulmonary and skin infections and eczema.

A **21.** **A.** false   **B.** false   **C.** false   **D.** true   **E.** true

The causes of neonatal vesicles include the common erythema toxicum neonatorum, and the rarer infantile acropustulosis.

Infectious causes include herpes simplex, bacterial sepsis and folliculitis.

A **22.** **A.** false **B.** false **C.** false **D.** false **E.** true

Alkaptonuria is due to a deficiency of homogentisic acid oxidase, resulting in homogentisic acid accumulating in the tissues and high levels appearing in the urine. Oxidation and polymerization of the homogentisic acid in the urine make it go dark on standing. The clinical features are ochronosis, a darkening of the tissues due to the accumulation of a black polymer of homogentisic acid in mesenchymal tissues. The other clinical features develop after puberty and are arthritis of the large joints and heart disease including heart valve calcification and myocardial infarction.

A **23.** **A.** false **B.** false **C.** true **D.** false **E.** false

Cystinosis is due to defective lysosomal transport of cystine. The early clinical features are due to Fanconi's syndrome. Cystinuria is a defect of renal proximal tubular reabsorption of the dibasic amino acids, causing renal stones and the complications associated with them (including hypertension).

A **24.** **A.** true **B.** false **C.** true **D.** true **E.** true

Glycogen storage diseases include GSDII (Pompe disease). The features are secondary to an inability to catabolize glycogen. Therefore during periods of starvation such as intercurrent illness, hypoglycaemia occurs. Hepatomegaly is due to the large quantities of glycogen stores. Long-term sequelae include osteoporosis, cardiac disease and short stature if untreated. They are managed with regular high-carbohydrate meals during the day, and continuous feeds during the night.

A **25.** **A.** false **B.** true **C.** false **D.** false **E.** false

Helicobacter pylori can increase or decrease gastric acid, hence when it is eradicated in some individuals acid production can actually increase compared to the preceding achlorhydria and the symptoms of gastro-oeseophageal reflux will worsen. Insulin-secreting β-cells of the pancreas have no measurable effect on gastic acid production. It is increased by vagal stimulation, gastrin release, histamine release affecting H2 receptors on oxyntic cells, and pepsin. It is decreased by low gastric pH, fear or sympathetic drive, and intestinal peptides such as cholesystokinin (pancreozymin), secretin, etc.

Murphey S, Aynsley-Green A, Wershil B. Chapter 4 and 5. In *Pediatric Gastrointestinal Disease*. Ed. Walker *et al*. St Louis: Mosby, 1996.

A 26. **A.** false   **B.** true   **C.** true   **D.** false   **E.** false

Lacteals are dilated and villi are distorted on small bowel biopsy. Faecal α-1-antitrypsin is a good marker of faecal protein loss and is therefore increased in intestinal lymphangiectasia. Learning difficulties and developmental regression occur in abetalipoproteinaemia.

A 27. **A.** true   **B.** true   **C.** false   **D.** true   **E.** true

Cullen's sign is a bluish periumbilical area seen in acute haemorrhagic pancreatitis.

Gaskin K. Chapter 29. In *Pediatric Gastrointestinal Disease*. Ed. Walker *et al*. St Louis: Mosby, 1996.

A 28. **A.** true   **B.** true   **C.** false   **D.** true   **E.** false

Recognized poor prognostic factors are: age under 10 years; shrinking liver size and falling transaminase levels; concomitant liver failure; paracetamol-induced liver failure; onset of liver failure less than 7 days from initial presentation. Consanguinity allows autosomal recessive conditions to surface but liver failure resulting from conditions such as tyrosinaemia or organic acidaemias do not have a worse prognosis than other causes.

Alonson E, Superina R, Whittington P. Chapter 5. In *Diseases of the Liver and Biliary System in Childhood*. Ed. Kelly D. Oxford: Blackwell Science, 1999.

A 29. **A.** true   **B.** true   **C.** false   **D.** false   **E.** true

With any tube inserted into the oesophagus and stomach, only the gastric balloon should be inflated as the flow is from the gastric fundus up to the oesophagus. Oesophageal pressure necrosis may otherwise result, and bleeding from fundal varices will be made worse. A Linton tube may be used, which only has a gastric balloon. Whereas lactulose may still play a part in removal of blood from the GI tract, there is now considered to be no place for the use of gut sterilization to prevent or diminish hepatic encephalopathy. The synthetic analogue of vasopressin, octreotide is useful in selectively decreasing splanchnic blood flow and portal pressure. It has also been described in other GI bleeding conditions as a temporizing measure.

Shepherd R. Chapter 11. In *Diseases of the Liver and Biliary System in Childhood*. Ed. Kelly D. Oxford: Blackwell Science, 1999.

A 30. A. true **B.** true **C.** false **D.** true **E.** true

A 31. A. false **B.** true **C.** false **D.** false **E.** true

Dilated cardiomyopathy affects predominantly the left venticle. A decreased ejection fraction is seen. Treatment includes anticoagulation to prevent embolism.

A 32. A. false **B.** true **C.** false **D.** false **E.** false

Prostaglandin E2 keeps the ductus arteriosus open in the first few days of life and is used for duct-dependent circulations (both systemic and pulmonary). Critical pulmonary stenosis and tricuspid atresia with intact ventricular septum both have duct-dependent pulmonary blood flow. Hypoplastic left heart syndrome and interrupted aortic arch have duct-dependent systemic circulations.

A 33. A. true **B.** false **C.** false **D.** true **E.** true

In atrial septal defect and mitral regurgitation there is a widely split second heart sound.

A 34. A. false **B.** false **C.** false **D.** false **E.** true

Ebstein's anomaly involves an abnormal tricuspid valve with leaflets adherent to the ventricular wall, a distally placed tricuspid valve, atrialization of the right ventricle, atrial septal defect, functional pulmonary atresia and Wolf-Parkinson-White (WPW) syndrome type B. Clinical symptoms include both SVT and extrasystoles.

A **35.** **A.** true **B.** false **C.** true **D.** false **E.** false

The urogenital ridges develop during the fifth
week of development. The ureteric bud gives rise to the ureter
and collecting ducts. The nephrogenic cap develops into
Bowman's capsules and the convoluted tubules.

A **36.** **A.** false **B.** true **C.** false **D.** true **E.** false

Classically, the large weight-bearing joints are affected by the
arthritis which is non-destructive. Thrombocytopenia is not a
feature. Approximately 15% of males have some form of
testicular involvement including epididymitis.

A **37.** **A.** false **B.** true **C.** false **D.** false **E.** false

Horseshoe kidney is present in 1 in 2000 people. The kidneys
are usually fused at the lower pole, and the ureters pass
anterior to the bridge.

A **38.** **A.** false **B.** false **C.** false **D.** false **E.** true

Post-streptococcal glomerulonephritis classically occurs 1–2
weeks after a Group A β-haemolytic Streptococcal
URTI. Renal biopsy is only indicated if there are unusual
features such as severe hypertension. Most cases will
spontaneously resolve, however microscopic haematuria can
continue in some cases.

A **39.** **A.** false **B.** false **C.** false **D.** false **E.** true

The cartilaginous tracheal rings develop from the
splanchnopleuric mesenchyme during the seventh week of
gestation. The lung buds develop in the fourth week of
gestation. Type II pneumocytes appear in the sixth month of
gestation. The trachea and oesophagus separate in the fourth
week of gestation.

A **40.** **A.** false **B.** true **C.** false **D.** false **E.** true

Lung surfactant is manufactured in type II pneumocytes in the
alveolar epithelium and is composed of phosphatidyl choline
(64%) and phosphatidyl glycerol (8%), with some other

proteins and lipids. It has an anti-atelectasis function by reducing surface tension at low lung volumes and increasing it at high volumes.

A **41.** **A.** true   **B.** false   **C.** true   **D.** true   **E.** false

The arthritis is very painful and often disproportionately so compared to the examination findings. The arthritis is fleeting, affecting individual joints for less than a week each, and it usually lasts less than 4 weeks altogether. Erythema marginatum is seen in less than 5% of cases.

A **42.** **A.** false   **B.** true   **C.** true   **D.** false   **E.** false

Malrotation is due to incomplete rotation of the intestine around the superior mesenteric artery in the third month of gestation. It can present as a protein-losing enteropathy secondary to bacterial overgrowth. It should always be treated surgically to avoid potential future serious consequences.

A **43.** **A.** true   **B.** true   **C.** true   **D.** true   **E.** false

Lamotrigine is used as monotherapy and adjunctive treatment of partial seizures and primary and secondarily generalized tonic-clonic seizures. Hepatic, renal and clotting parameters should be closely monitored, as hepatic dysfunction and bone marrow failure may occur.

A **44.** **A.** true   **B.** true   **C.** false   **D.** false   **E.** false

Penicillamine can cause nephrotic syndrome, dermatomyositis, SLE-like syndrome and haemolytic anaemia.

A **45.** **A.** true   **B.** true   **C.** false   **D.** false   **E.** true

Zero-order kinetics occur when the enzyme responsible for the reaction is saturated. The rate of elimination varies with the plasma concentration.
The absolute amount eliminated is the same regardless of plasma concentration. A constant amount of drug is metabolized per unit time.

A **46.** **A.** true **B.** false **C.** true **D.** false **E.** true

Children with Asperger's syndrome have variable fine and gross motor delay. They have no language delay, but have unusual language development (e.g. tend to interpret literally, and have one-sided conversations). They also have difficulty comprehending non-verbal communication.

A **47.** **A.** true **B.** true **C.** false **D.** false **E.** true

The carbon dioxide response curve is shifted to the left in neonates (i.e. they have a decreased ventilatory response to hypercarbia). The physiological dead space is about one-third of the tidal volume, as in adults. The airways are narrow and therefore have a higher resistance.

A **48.** **A.** true **B.** false **C.** false **D.** true **E.** true

Congenital lobar emphysema usually presents in the neonatal period with severe respiratory distress, though in a minority of cases, symptoms are not apparent until a few months (or rarely a few years) of age. The left upper lobe is the most frequently affected. It is associated with tetralogy of Fallot and anomalous left pulmonary artery. Treatment is with selective ventilation and/or lobectomy.

A **49.** **A.** true **B.** true **C.** true **D.** false **E.** true

Nitric oxide diffuses to arteriolar smooth muscle cells where it activates guanyl cyclase to convert guanosine triphosphate (GTP) to cyclic guanosine monophosphate (cGMP), which causes pulmonary arteriolar smooth muscle relaxation. Nitric oxide is inactivated by binding to haemoglobin and forming nitrosohaemoglobin and methaemoglobin.

A **50.** **A.** false **B.** true **C.** true **D.** false **E.** true

Increased maternal serum alpha-fetoprotein is seen in multiple pregnancy, anencephaly, open spina bifida, anterior abdominal wall defects, Turner syndrome, cystic hygroma, renal agenesis, polycystic kidneys and hereditary persistence. Trisomy 18 causes a decrease in maternal serum alpha-fetoprotein.

51. **A.** true **B.** true **C.** true **D.** false **E.** false

Linoleic and linolenic acid are essential fatty acids. Essential amino acids for the preterm neonate are leucine, isoleucine, valine, threonine, methionine, phenylalanine, tryptophan and lysine.

A **52.** **A.** false **B.** false **C.** false **D.** false **E.** true

In type 1 diabetes 80% of children have islet cell antibodies on presentation. The risk of developing the disease is 1 in 20 for siblings, 1 in 20 if the father is affected and 1 in 40 if the mother is affected. Identical twin concordance is over 80%. The current prevalence in the UK is 1 in 300 and rising.

A **53.** **A.** true **B.** true **C.** true **D.** false **E.** false

Intracranial pathology can cause SIADH by increasing the secretion of ADH due to local effects, and intrathoracic pathology can cause it by stimulating volume receptors. Drugs that cause SIADH include morphine, carbamazepine, chlorpropamide, vincristine, vinblastin and cyclophosphamide. Lithium and demeclocycline can both cause renal diabetes insipidus.

A **54.** **A.** true **B.** true **C.** true **D.** false **E.** false

Autoimmune polyendocrine syndrome type II is the association of chronic lymphocytic thyroiditis, diabetes mellitus and adrenal insufficiency.

A **55.** **A.** true **B.** true **C.** false **D.** false **E.** false

Hypothyroidism, testicular feminization syndrome and the empty sella syndrome are all causes of primary amenorrhoea with secondary sexual characteristics.

A **56.** **A.** false **B.** true **C.** false **D.** true **E.** false

Delayed puberty is defined in girls as failure of onset of any signs of puberty by age 13 years, and by age 14 years in boys. It may be caused by congenital adrenal hyperplasia due to 3β-hydroxysteroid dehydrogenase deficiency. It is most common in boys, usually due to constitutional delay.

Exam 4

Answers

A 57. **A.** false   **B.** false   **C.** false   **D.** false   **E.** false

The contraindications to pertussis vaccination are general considerations (acute febrile illness or anaphylaxis to previous dose), and children with an evolving neurological problem. In children with a stable neurological condition, there is no contraindication.

A 58. **A.** false   **B.** false   **C.** false   **D.** true   **E.** false

Diphtheria is caused by *Corynebacterium diphtheriae*, of which the gravis type causes the most severe disease, then intermedius, with mitis causing the mildest disease. The disease is toxin-induced with subunit A causing the clinical disease and subunit B transporting the toxin to target receptors. The incubation period is short, from 2 to 7 days. Where diphtheria is endemic, an estimated 2–5% of healthy individuals harbour the organism.

A 59. **A.** false   **B.** false   **C.** true   **D.** true   **E.** true

Otitis media is usually bacterial in origin, of which the most common infective agent is *Streptococcus pneumoniae*, then *Moxarella catarrhalis* and *Haemophilus influenzae*. Two weeks following an episode of acute otitis media, approximately 70% of children will have an effusion, falling to around 20% at 1 month. These children will have consequent temporary hearing impairment.

A 60. **A.** false   **B.** false   **C.** false   **D.** true   **E.** true

Lymphadenitis is most commonly due to *Staphylococcus aureus* infection, then Group A β-haemolytic Streptococcal infection. In mycobacterium infection, the lymphadenopathy is non-tender.

Q 1. **The following genetic conditions are associated with congenital limb hemihypertrophy**

    A. Russell-Silver syndrome
    B. Conradi-Hunermann syndrome
    C. Neurofibromatosis
    D. Marfan syndrome
    E. CHILD syndrome

Q 2. **Regarding the Potter sequence**

    A. It is a disruption sequence
    B. Clubbed feet are a feature
    C. It may be secondary to prolonged rupture of membranes
    D. It is associated with breech presentation
    E. Parents should have a renal ultrasound scan

Q 3. **Lip pits**

    A. Are part of Van der Woude syndrome
    B. Derive from accessory salivary glands
    C. Are associated with missing incisors
    D. Are associated with cleft lip and palate
    E. Are of autosomal recessive inheritance

Q 4. **Iris colobomas are associated with**

    A. Trisomy 13
    B. 4p-syndrome
    C. 13q-syndrome
    D. Goltz syndrome
    E. CHARGE association

Q 5. **The following definitions are correct**

    A. Clinodactyly – curvature of a digit due to hypoplasia of the middle phalynx

B. Syndactyly – incomplete separation of digits
C. Camptodactyly – abnormally wide girth of digits
D. Mesomelia – relative shortness of upper arms
E. Hypertelorism – abnormally widely spaced medial canthi

Q 6. **In benign intracranial hypertension**

A. The cerebral ventricles may be small
B. There is elevated CSF protein
C. It may be caused by hypothyroidism
D. 90% of cases are idiopathic
E. It may be caused by nitrofurantoin

Q 7. **The following CSF findings and metabolic conditions are associated**

A. Low CSF protein – Metachromatic leukodystrophy
B. CSF Glycine – Non-ketotic hyperglycinaemia
C. CSF Glycine – Pyridoxine deficiency
D. Low CSF lactate – Menkes syndrome
E. High CSF lactate – Mitochondrial disorders

Q 8. **A VIIth nerve palsy in a child may be due to**

A. Moebius sequence
B. Williams syndrome
C. Ramsay Hunt syndrome
D. Lyme disease
E. Varicella infection

Q 9. **Vertigo secondary to vestibular nerve or labyrinthine dysfunction will be associated with**

A. No hearing loss
B. Tinnitus
C. Falls away from the direction of unilateral disease
D. Nystagmus
E. Ataxia if bilateral disease

Q 10. **The following can cause pinpoint pupils**

A. Pontine lesions
B. Organophosphates

C. Barbiturates
D. Nutmeg poisoning
E. Morphine

Q 11. **The following developmental features would raise concern of possible cerebral palsy**

A. Head lag persisting beyond 2 months
B. Inability to crawl by 8 months
C. Inability to sit straight by 6 months
D. Inability to bring the hands together in the midline while supine by 4 months
E. Hand dominance present at 6 months

Q 12. **A child being developmentally assessed is able to unbutton his front buttons, stand briefly on one foot and ride a tricycle. This corresponds to a developmental age in a normal child of**

A. 2.5 years
B. 2 years
C. 4 years
D. 3.5 years
E. 3 years

Q 13. **Regarding retinopathy of prematurity**

A. It should be screened for in any neonate under 1800 g birth weight
B. Normal retinal vasculature begins to develop from 8 weeks in utero
C. It is a cause of retinal detachment
D. It should be treated if stage 2 disease
E. It can be treated with cryotherapy

Q 14. **The following are ocular features of Waardenburg syndrome**

A. Optic atrophy
B. Retinal hypopigmentation
C. Confluent eyebrows
D. Iris heterochromia
E. Strabismus

Q 15. **Acute inflammation can cause the following changes in blood tests**

A. Elevated platelet count
B. Decreased transferrin saturation
C. A raised serum transferrin level
D. A raised serum iron level
E. A reduction in ferritin level

Q 16. **Pyruvate kinase (PK) deficiency**

A. Most commonly affects Mediterranean people
B. Usually presents with symptoms of profound anaemia
C. Causes a left shift of the oxyhaemoglobin dissociation curve
D. Is a cause of renal stones
E. Is a cause of splenomegaly

Q 17. **In Glucose-6-phosphate dehydrogenase (G6PD) deficiency type B**

A. The young red blood cells are unaffected
B. Haemolytic episodes are usually self-limiting
C. It is seen in Afro-Caribbeans
D. Viral infections may trigger haemolytic episodes
E. Howell-Jolly bodies are present in a crisis

Q 18. **Causes of finger clubbing include**

A. Hypothyroidism
B. Small bowel lymphoma
C. Congenital methaemoglobinaemia
D. Idiopathic
E. Familial

Q 19. **In autoimmune haemolytic anaemia caused by 'warm' antibodies**

A. The antibodies are IgM
B. The haemolysis is mostly intravascular
C. It is associated with *Mycoplasma pneumoniae* infection
D. Chronic haemolysis is unlikely
E. Steroids are usually ineffective

Q 20. **Humoral immunodeficiency disorders are characterized by infections with**

A. *Candida albicans*
B. *Giardia lamblia*

C. *Aspergillus*

D. Enteroviruses

E. *Mycoplasma*

Q 21. Skin prick testing is affected by

A. A child's age

B. Season

C. Body site

D. Steroid medication

E. A child's sex

Q 22. Neonatal hyperammonaemia is seen in

A. Fatty acid oxidation defects

B. Hereditary fructose intolerance

C. Neonatal haemochromatosis

D. Urea cycle defects

E. Propionic acidaemia

Q 23. The following are features of Wilson's disease

A. It is a cause of distal renal tubular acidosis

B. The gene defect is on chromosome 7

C. Urinary copper excretion is decreased

D. It is a cause of haemolytic anaemia

E. It may present with convulsions

Q 24. Peroxisomal biogenesis disorders

A. Are characterized by dysmorphic features

B. May show chondrodysplasia punctata on X-ray

C. Are a cause of corneal clouding

D. Are characterized by elevated very long chain fatty acids

E. Include Smith-Lemni-Opitz syndrome

Q 25. In paediatric orthoptic liver transplant

A. Generalized mitochondrial cytopathy is a recognized indication

B. The major indication in Alagille's syndrome is deteriorating liver synthetic function

C. The host liver is left *in situ*

D. CMV status of host and recipient is unimportant

E. 5-year survival rate for an elective transplant is 80–90%

Q 26. **When liver pathology is responsible for an acutely ill baby**

    A. Intraocular 'oildrop' cataracts point towards galactosaemia as the diagnosis

    B. Blood and urine should always be taken and stored at $-70\,^{\circ}C$ if hypoglycaemia is present

    C. Hyperlactaemia excludes mitochondrial cytopathies

    D. Bile-stained vomiting points towards biliary atresia

    E. Intragastric infusion of ursodeoxycholic acid is important in the initial management

Q 27. **Hepatic glycogen storage disorders**

    A. Display autosomal recessive inheritance

    B. Characteristically show a low cholesterol and raised triglycerides

    C. Cause hepatosplenomegaly from birth

    D. Frequently cause cataracts

    E. Management consists of stem cell transplantation, with or without liver transplantation

Q 28. **Crohn's disease is more likely if**

    A. There is rectal sparing

    B. An anal tag is present

    C. Non-specific gastritis is seen on upper endoscopy

    D. Strictures are seen in the transverse colon

    E. Fever, malaise and lethargy are present

Q 29. **Acute pancreatitis in childhood**

    A. May be caused by the use of total parenteral nutrition

    B. Can cause a right pleural effusion

    C. Is associated with Kawasaki disease

    D. Causes hypercalcaemia

    E. Occurs in myasthenia gravis

Q 30. **A loud first heart sound occurs in**

    A. Impaired left ventricular function

    B. Obesity

    C. Fever

    D. Mitral stenosis

    E. Transposition of the great arteries

Q 31. The following are recognized manifestations of ostium secundum atrial septal defect

- **A.** Apical ejection click
- **B.** Parasternal thrill
- **C.** Mid-diastolic tricuspid flow murmur
- **D.** Fixed wide splitting of the second heart sound
- **E.** Left axis deviation

Q 32. Mitral valve prolapse is a feature of

- **A.** Neurofibromatosis
- **B.** Osteogenesis imperfecta
- **C.** Noonan syndrome
- **D.** Klinefelter's syndrome
- **E.** Hurler syndrome

Q 33. Maternal diabetes mellitus is associated with the following neonatal cardiac conditions

- **A.** Congenital heart block
- **B.** Aortic stenosis
- **C.** Pericarditis
- **D.** Transposition of the great arteries
- **E.** Ebstein's anomaly

Q 34. The following conditions cause increased pulmonary vascular markings on chest X-ray

- **A.** Transposition of the great arteries
- **B.** Tetralogy of Fallot
- **C.** Truncus arteriosus
- **D.** Ebstein's anomaly
- **E.** Pulmonary atresia

Q 35. Regarding development of the urogenital system

- **A.** The loops of Henle develop after birth
- **B.** Bowman's capsules start to form in the fourth week
- **C.** The glomerular filtration membrane is functional from the third trimester
- **D.** The collecting ductules develop from the third month in utero
- **E.** Unilateral renal agenesis is present in 1 in 2000 individuals

Q 36. **The following conditions can cause hyperkalaemia in children**

    A. Hyperaldosteronism
    B. Proximal renal tubular acidosis
    C. Exercise
    D. Chemotherapy
    E. Trauma

Q 37. **Regarding asymptomatic haematuria**

    A. It is more common in boys
    B. It may be caused by hypercalciuria
    C. If associated with proteinuria it may be due to benign familial haematuria
    D. It may be caused by sickle cell anaemia
    E. It is a feature of Berger's nephropathy

Q 38. **The following conditions are likely to progress to chronic renal impairment**

    A. Alport syndrome
    B. Berger's nephropathy
    C. Minimal change nephritic syndrome
    D. Diabetes mellitus
    E. Post-streptococcal glomerulonephritis

Q 39. **Regarding the sinuses**

    A. The maxillary and ethmoid sinuses develop from 6 months of age
    B. The sphenoid sinus is present from birth
    C. The frontal sinus develops from 3 to 7 years of age
    D. Approximately 25% of the population have no frontal sinus
    E. Allergic rhinitis predisposes to chronic sinusitis

Q 40. **The following conditions are associated with nasal polyps**

    A. Bronchiolitis
    B. Malignancy
    C. Allergic rhinitis
    D. Kartagener's syndrome
    E. Thalassaemia

Q 41. **A 5-year-old girl with chronic asthma, presenting with fever, eosinophilia and a purpuric rash and with necrotizing vasculitis on skin biopsy could be diagnosed with**

    A. Polyarteritis nodosa
    B. Wegener's granulomatosis
    C. Henoch-Schönlein purpura
    D. Churg-Strauss syndrome
    E. Goodpasture's disease

Q 42. **An 18-month-old boy with bilateral impalpable undescended testes lying along the normal line of descent should be managed with**

    A. Unilateral orchidectomy with counterside orchidectomy 6 months later
    B. MRI scan to locate them and then follow up to see if they descend by age 2 years
    C. Examination under anaesthesia or laparoscopy to locate them and then orchidopexy
    D. Karyotype and then observation
    E. Initial serial HCG injections

Q 43. **The following drugs exhibit substantial hepatic first-pass metabolism**

    A. Verapamil
    B. Hydralazine
    C. Alcohol
    D. Labetalol
    E. Codeine

Q 44. **Vigabatrin**

    A. Is a GABA transaminase inhibitor
    B. Is given for infantile spasms
    C. Causes dose-independent excitation in children
    D. Causes central retinal atrophy
    E. Causes rickets

Q 45. **Ciclosporin**

    A. Is a non-calcineurin inhibiting immunosuppressant
    B. Is myelotoxic

C. Is used for treating graft-versus-host disease
D. Can cause gout
E. May cause myalgia

Q 46. **The following are associated with faecal soiling**

A. Marital breakdown
B. Learning difficulties
C. Hypothyroidism
D. Hirschsprung's disease
E. Anal fissure

Q 47. **The following drugs may adversely affect the fetus when given to the mother during the last 4 weeks of pregnancy**

A. Isotretinoin
B. Cocaine
C. Warfarin
D. Paracetamol
E. Phenoxymethylpenicillin

Q 48. **Regarding thermoregulation in neonates**

A. Neonates have a lower density of sweat glands than adults
B. Neonatal sweat response to thermal stimuli is equal to that of adults
C. Brown fat lipolysis is stimulated by noradrenaline and thyroid hormone
D. Brown fat stores are located in the intrascapular and axillary regions
E. Muscular activity is used to generate heat

Q 49. **The following classically cause vomiting during the first week of life**

A. Meconium ileus
B. Duodenal atresia
C. Pyloric stenosis
D. Hiatus hernia
E. Malrotation

Fetal haemoglobin

A. Binds more easily to 2,3-DPG than adult haemoglobin
B. Has a lower affinity for oxygen than adult haemoglobin (HbA)
C. Forms approximately 60% of haemoglobin at birth
D. Is made up of two alpha and two delta chains
E. Is present in thalassaemia intermedia syndrome

Q 51. Maternal breast milk for preterm infants compared to that for full-term infants

A. Has the same composition
B. Has a higher protein content
C. Has a higher calorific content
D. Is higher in carbohydrates
E. Is higher in trace elements

Q 52. Plasma calcium levels are elevated in

A. Hypoparathyroidism
B. Fanconi's syndrome
C. Vitamin D resistant rickets
D. Secondary hyperparathyroidism
E. Pseudohypoparathyroidism

Q 53. Thyroxine

A. Contributes to skeletal growth
B. Is predominantly albumin-bound in the plasma
C. Is 20% free in the plasma
D. Cannot cross the placenta
E. Levels may be normal in the sick euthyroid syndrome

Q 54. The anterior pituitary gland secretes

A. Somatostatin
B. Follicle-stimulating hormone
C. Growth hormone
D. Oxytocin
E. Thyrotrophin-releasing hormone

Q 55. The following are associated with neonatal micropenis

A. Kallman syndrome
B. Maternal cocaine use during the second trimester

C. Maternal diabetes mellitus
D. Sotos syndrome
E. Septo-optic dysplasia

Q 56. The following are true of hormonal tests used in growth disorders

A. Random growth hormone levels are usually low during the daytime in children
B. IGF-1 levels may be high in malnutrition
C. IGF-1 levels are a good indication of growth hormone status
D. IGF-binding protein-3 (IGFBP-3) levels are less affected by nutritional factors than IGF-1
E. Somatomedin 3 is unhelpful in assessing short stature

Q 57. Varicella zoster virus vaccine

A. Should be given to children receiving radiotherapy
B. Should be given to children on long-term high-dose oral steroids
C. Cannot be given during pregnancy
D. Should be given to a newborn infant whose mother developed chicken pox 2 days prior to delivery
E. Should be given to children with hypogammaglobulinaemia

Q 58. Cat scratch disease

A. Is due to *Coxiella burnetii* infection
B. Causes regional non-tender lymphadenitis
C. Is a cause of arthralgia
D. May result in granulomatous lesion in the liver
E. May enter via the eye

Q 59. The following infective agents can cause a clinical presentation mimicking infectious mononucleosis

A. *Bartonella henselae*
B. Adenovirus
C. Rubella
D. Cytomegalovirus
E. *Giardia*

Infections associated with the production of atypical lymphocytes include

    A. Rubella

    B. Mumps

    C. Roseola infantum

    D. Tuberculosis

    E. Toxoplasmosis

A 1.   **A.** true   **B.** true   **C.** true   **D.** false   **E.** true

Congenital limb hemihypertrophy is seen in Russell-Silver syndrome, Conradi-Hunermann syndrome, neurofibromatosis, Proteus syndrome and CHILD syndrome.

A 2.   **A.** false   **B.** true   **C.** true   **D.** true   **E.** true

Parents of infants with Potter syndrome secondary to renal agenesis should have a renal ultrasound scan as it can be of autosomal dominant inheritance with variable expression resulting in unilateral renal agenesis in a parent. Potter syndrome is a deformation sequence. Potter sequence is a pattern of fetal malformations caused by extreme oligohydramnios. The underlying problem is classically renal agenesis, however other causes of oligohydramnios including prolonged rupture of membranes can cause the same sequence.

A 3.   **A.** true   **B.** true   **C.** false   **D.** true   **E.** false

Lip pits are associated with both cleft lip and palate and missing second premolars as part of the Van der Woude syndrome. The inheritance is autosomal dominant with variable expression.

A 4.   **A.** true   **B.** true   **C.** true   **D.** true   **E.** true

If iris colobomas are present, chromosomal analysis is advisable.

A 5.   **A.** true   **B.** true   **C.** false   **D.** false   **E.** false

Camptodactyly is abnormal persistent flexion of digits. Mesomelia means relative shortness of forearms. Hypertelorism is abnormally widely spaced interpupillary distance.

A 6.   **A.** true   **B.** false   **C.** false   **D.** true   **E.** true

In benign intracranial hypertension there is a raised CSF pressure with an otherwise normal CSF profile. The ventricles are usually normal size but may be small. There are many causes including drugs (e.g. steroids, tetracyclines, oral contraceptive pill), hormonal (e.g. hypoparathyroidism and pseudohypoparathyroidism) and pregnancy.

A7. **A.** false **B.** true **C.** true **D.** false **E.** true

In metachromatic leukodystrophy there is a raised CSF protein. In Menkes syndrome there is a raised CSF lactate.

A8. **A.** true **B.** false **C.** true **D.** true **E.** true

The Moebius sequence involves a mask-like facies with VIth and VIIth nerve palsy (usually bilateral) secondary to various mechanisms.

A9. **A.** false **B.** true **C.** false **D.** true **E.** true

Vertigo secondary to vestibular nerve or labyrinthine dysfunction is *peripheral* vertigo and is associated with hearing loss. Falls are in the direction of unilateral disease. Central vertigo would be caused by abnormalities of the CNS (temporal lobe or brain stem).

A10. **A.** true **B.** true **C.** true **D.** true **E.** true

Pinpoint pupils result from an imbalance between the constricting parasympathetic nervous system (accompanying the IIIrd cranial nerve) and the dilating sympathetic nerve fibres (ciliary nerve). Structural lesions in the pons affect the sympathetic fibres.

A11. **A.** false **B.** false **C.** false **D.** true **E.** true

Head lag persisting beyond 6 months and inability to sit straight by 8 months (normal infants can sit with a bent back at 6 months) are abnormal. Obvious hand dominance before 1 year of age should alert one to the possibility of cerebral palsy, but needs to be taken in context with other clinical signs. The age at which infants crawl is very variable, but inability to crawl by one year (in the absence of walking or bottom-shuffling) is abnormal.

A12. **A.** false **B.** false **C.** false **D.** false **E.** true

A13. **A.** false **B.** false **C.** true **D.** false **E.** true

Retinopathy of prematurity is screened for in infants under 1500 g or 32 weeks' gestation. The normal retinal vasculature develops from 16 weeks' gestation. Stage 3 disease and above are treated. It can be treated using laser or cryotherapy.

A **14.** **A.** false **B.** true **C.** true **D.** true **E.** false

The ocular features of Waardenburg syndrome are: lateral displacement of the inner canthi (type I), short palpebral fissures, medial flare of bushy eyebrows which may be confluent, retinal hypopigmentation and heterochromic iris.

A **15.** **A.** true **B.** true **C.** false **D.** false **E.** false

Ferritin levels rise, and serum transferrin levels and serum iron levels decrease.

A **16.** **A.** false **B.** false **C.** false **D.** false **E.** true

Pyruvate kinase deficiency affects people worldwide. Whilst the anaemia may be quite profound, the symptoms are relatively mild due to the right shift of the oxyhaemoglobin dissociation curve secondary to compensatory increase in 2,3 DPG levels. It is a cause of gallstones and splenomegaly.

A **17.** **A.** false **B.** false **C.** false **D.** true **E.** false

Glucose-6-phosphate dehydrogenase (G6PD) deficiency type B is the more severe Mediterranean type, in which all the red cells including reticulocytes have reduced enzyme activity. Haemolytic episodes therefore are severe. Features of intravascular haemolysis are seen on the blood film during a crisis including bite cells, blister cells and Heinz bodies.

A **18.** **A.** true **B.** true **C.** true **D.** true **E.** true

The causes of finger clubbing may be divided into any cause of chronic cyanosis (respiratory, cardiovascular or other), gastrointestinal and liver disorders, and endocrine disorders. It may also be a variant of normal; either inherited or sporadic idiopathic.

A **19.** **A.** false **B.** false **C.** false **D.** false **E.** false

In haemolytic anaemia caused by 'warm' antibodies the antibodies are usually IgG and have best activity at 37 °C. The haemolysis is mostly extravascular due to consumption within the spleen. The causes are often underlying chronic disorders including autoimmune diseases, haematological malignancies and drugs, and so it may become chronic. Steroids are often effective treatment.

A **20.** **A.** false **B.** true **C.** false **D.** true **E.** true

Defects of humoral immunity manifest with the following:
Bacterial infections: staphylococci, streptococci, *Haemophilus influenzae*, *Moxarella catarrhalis*, *Mycoplasma* and *Campylobacter*
Viral infections: Enteroviruses
Protozoal infections: *Giardia lamblia*

A **21.** **A.** true **B.** true **C.** true **D.** true **E.** false

The wheal reaction is less in an infant, and begins to decrease again from around age 50 years. Different sites of the body have different reactivity to allergens, and therefore a specific site needs to be used for uniformity of results. Skin prick testing is usually performed on the medial forearm. Both steroid and antihistamine medication can suppress skin prick reactions.

A **22.** **A.** true **B.** false **C.** true **D.** true **E.** true

The main groups of metabolic diseases that cause neonatal hyperammonaemia are fatty acid oxidation defects, urea cycle defects and organic acidaemias.

A **23.** **A.** false **B.** false **C.** false **D.** true **E.** true

Wilson's disease is caused by a copper transport defect, the gene is mapped to chromosome 13q14–21. Urine copper excretion is high. The features include a proximal renal tubular acidosis.

A **24.** **A.** true **B.** true **C.** true **D.** true **E.** false

Smith-Lemni-Opitz syndrome is caused by an enzyme defect in the synthesis of cholesterol.

A **25.** **A.** false **B.** false **C.** false **D.** false **E.** true

Multisystem involvement is usual with mitochondrial cytopathies, especially when uncovered by fulminant liver failure with sodium valproate treatment, and is a direct contraindication to liver transplant as the child will unfortunately die from irreversible neurological deterioration despite a normally functioning liver graft. The major indication in Alagille's syndrome is poor quality of life due to intense pruritis. The host liver is virtually never left *in situ* as the hepatic artery and vein and portal vein are utilized for the donor organ. The chance of post-transplant CMV infection in an immunocompromised individual is highest if the donor is CMV positive, and less so if the recipient is negative.

Kelly D, Ayer D. Chapter 17. In *Diseases of the Liver and Biliary System in Childhood*. Ed. Kelly D. Oxford: Blackwell Science, 1999.

A **26.** **A.** true **B.** true **C.** false **D.** false **E.** false

LFTs will normalize within days of removal of galactose from the diet in galactosaemia. Reducing substances may be present in the urine in other infant disorders. Conversely, galactosuria may not occur if no lactose or galactose is present in the diet. Lactate is almost always raised to above 5 mmol/L in mitochondrial cytopathies. Occasionally, choledochal cysts can be large enough to cause intestinal obstruction and bile-stained vomiting, but this does not occur in biliary atresia. Oral ursodeoxycholic acid (a synthetic bile acid inducing cholorhesis) may help in the prevention of chronic cholestasis (e.g. in cystic fibrosis or TPN-associated cholestasis), but is not helpful in the acute situation.

McKiernan P, Roberts E, Kelly D. Chapter 3. In *Diseases of the Liver and Biliary System in Childhood*. Ed. Kelly D. Oxford: Blackwell Science, 1999.

A **27.** **A.** true **B.** false **C.** false **D.** false **E.** false

Characteristically, cholesterol is raised >6 mmol/L, triglycerides >3 mmol/L, uric acid is raised >350 mmol/L, lactate >5 mmol/L, aminotransferases may be mildly low <2.5 mmol/L, but bilirubin, albumin and coagulation are normal. Cataracts occur in mucopolysaccharidoses. Lipid storage disorders cause both liver and spleen to be enlarged, but glycogen storage disorders affect the liver only. Nephromegaly may occur in Type Ia.

Liver transplant may be required in Types III and IV, and rarely for Type Ia if symptomatic multiple hepatic adenomas occur, or to prevent hepatocellular carcinoma. Bone marrow transplant is useful for some lipid storage disorders but not glycogen storage disorders.

Green A, Kelly D. Chapter 9. In *Diseases of the Liver and Biliary System in Childhood.* Ed. Kelly D. Oxford: Blackwell Science, 1999.

A 28. A. true **B.** true **C.** false **D.** false **E.** false

Non-specific gastritis can occur in ulcerative colitis as well as Crohn's disease. Colonic strictures can occur in both conditions. Non-specific symptoms occur in both, although malnutrition can have a slightly increased prevalence in Crohn's disease, and ulcerative colitis is the more likely diagnosis if PR bleeding is present.

Leichtner A, Jackson W, Grand R. Chapter 27. In *Pediatric Gastrointestinal Disease.* Ed. Walker A *et al.* St Louis: Mosby, 1996.

A 29. A. true **B.** true **C.** true **D.** false **E.** false

A left pleural effusion occurs more often than on the right. Hypocalcaemia is common.

Sidwell RU, Thomson M. *Concise Paediatrics.* London: Greenwich Medical Media Ltd., 2000.

A 30. A. false **B.** false **C.** true **D.** true **E.** false

Conditions that increase the cardiac output cause a loud first heart sound, including fever, exercise and thyrotoxicosis.

A 31. A. false **B.** false **C.** true **D.** true **E.** false

In an ostium secundum ASD, the murmur is ejection systolic in the upper left sternal edge. There may also be a mid-diastolic tricuspid flow murmur at the lower left sternal edge due to increased tricuspid flow. The ECG shows *right* axis deviation, a partial *right* bundle branch block (in 90%) and *right* ventricular hypertrophy. Left axis deviation or a superior axis is seen in an ostium primum defect.

A 32. A. false **B.** true **C.** false **D.** false **E.** true

Mitral valve prolapse is seen in connective tissue disorders including Marfan syndrome, certain forms of Ehlers-Danlos syndrome and pseudoxanthoma elasticum.

A 33. A. false **B.** true **C.** false **D.** true **E.** false

Diabetes mellitus is associated with neonatal VSD, transposition of the great arteries and left ventricular outflow obstruction (aortic stenosis and septal hypertrophy).

A 34. A. true **B.** false **C.** true **D.** false **E.** false

Tetralogy of Fallot, Ebstein's anomaly and pulmonary atresia cause pulmonary oligaemia on chest X-ray.

A 35. A. true **B.** false **C.** false **D.** true **E.** false

Bowman's capsules start to form in the eighth week of gestation. The glomerular filtration membrane is functional from the second trimester. Unilateral renal agenesis is present in 1 in 1000 individuals.

A 36. A. false **B.** false **C.** true **D.** true **E.** true

Hyperaldosteronism and proximal renal tubular acidosis causes hypokalaemia. Exercise, chemotherapy and trauma increase catabolism, which moves potassium into the circulation from the cells.

A 37. A. false **B.** true **C.** false **D.** true **E.** true

Asymptomatic haematuria is more common in girls.

A 38. A. true **B.** true **C.** false **D.** true **E.** false

Renal failure develops in Alport syndrome by age 20–30 years. 25% of patients with Berger's nephropathy eventually develop chronic renal failure.

A 39. A. false **B.** false **C.** true **D.** false **E.** true

The maxillary and ethmoid sinuses are present from birth. The sphenoid sinus develops from 2 to 3 years of age. Approximately 10% of the population have no frontal sinus.

A 40. A. false   **B.** true   **C.** true   **D.** true   **E.** false

Nasal polyps are also associated with cystic fibrosis and chronic sinusitis.

A 41. A. false   **B.** false   **C.** false   **D.** true   **E.** false

A 42. A. false   **B.** false   **C.** true   **D.** false   **E.** false

A 43. A. true   **B.** true   **C.** false   **D.** true   **E.** true

Drugs which have a significant hepatic first-pass metabolism include: verapamil, isosorbide dinitrate, glyceryl trinitrate, hydralazine, propanolol, labetalol, aspirin, codeine and morphine.

A 44. A. true   **B.** true   **C.** false   **D.** false   **E.** false

Vigabatrin causes peripheral retinal atrophy. The excitation seen in children disappears with dose reduction.

A 45. A. false   **B.** false   **C.** true   **D.** true   **E.** true

Ciclosporin is a calcineurin inhibitor. It is virtually non-myelotoxic, but is markedly nephrotoxic (dose-dependent). Renal function and blood pressure therefore need to be closely monitored, particularly during the first few weeks of use. Other side-effects are gingival hypertrophy and hypertrichosis.

A 46. A. true   **B.** true   **C.** true   **D.** true   **E.** true

The causes of faecal soiling can be divided into:

Children with normal bowel control with soiling in response to stress only.
Faecal retention with overflow incontinence (e.g. anal fissure causing painful defecation then constipation, hypothyroidism and Hirschsprung's disease).
Neurological damage causing a failure to establish bowel control.

A **47.** **A.** true **B.** true **C.** true **D.** false **E.** false

Warfarin can cause fetal malformations, particularly between 6 and 9 weeks, and fetal haemorrhage in the second and third trimesters. Cocaine can cause placental abruption, intracranial haemorrhage and premature delivery.

A **48.** **A.** false **B.** true **C.** true **D.** true **E.** true

In a cold environment, the sympathetic nervous system is stimulated, inducing the release of noradrenaline and thyroid hormone which cause lipolysis of brown fats. There are brown fat stores in the intrascapular and axillary, mediastinal, perirenal, paraspinal and nuchal regions. Neonatal sweat response to thermal stimuli is one-third less than that of adults.

A **49.** **A.** true **B.** true **C.** false **D.** true **E.** true

Pyloric stenosis classically causes vomiting at 6 weeks of age.

A **50.** **A.** false **B.** false **C.** false **D.** false **E.** false

Fetal haemoglobin is composed of two alpha and two gamma chains and forms over 80% of haemoglobin at birth. It binds less easily to 2,3-DPG than adult haemoglobin, therefore the oxyhaemoglobin curve is shifted to the left, and it has a higher affinity for oxygen than adult haemoglobin. Thalassaemia intermedia is an α thalassaemia in which there is HbH, HbA and Hb Barts.

A **51.** **A.** false **B.** true **C.** true **D.** false **E.** true

Maternal breast milk for preterm infants compared to that for full-term infants has a higher protein, calorie and lipid content and lower carbohydrate content. It is also higher in many minerals, trace elements and vitamins (especially A and E).

A **52.** **A.** false **B.** false **C.** false **D.** false **E.** false

In hypoparathyroidism, vitamin D resistant rickets, secondary hyperparathyroidism and psuedohypoparathyroidism, plasma calcium levels are low. In Fanconi's syndrome they are normal.

A. true **B.** false **C.** false **D.** false **E.** true

Thyroxine is 99.98% protein-bound in the circulation. It binds to thyroxine-binding globulin (predominantly), thyroxine-binding prealbumin and albumin. In the sick euthyroid syndrome T3 is low, T4 may be low or normal and the TSH level is normal or low. It occurs in acute or chronic illness.

A 54. **A.** false **B.** true **C.** true **D.** false **E.** false

The anterior pituitary secretes growth hormone, ACTH, luteinizing hormone (LH), follicle-stimulating hormone (FSH), thyroid stimulating-hormone (TSH) and prolactin.

A 55. **A.** true **B.** false **C.** false **D.** false **E.** true

Kallman syndrome and septo-optic dysplasia, CHARGE association, Noonan syndrome and Prader-Willi syndrome are all associated with neonatal micropenis.

A 56. **A.** true **B.** false **C.** true **D.** true **E.** false

Because random growth hormone levels are usually low during the daytime in children they are not useful in assessing short stature. Instead, insulin growth factor-1 (IGF-1) and IGF-binding protein-3 (IGFBP-3) levels are looked at to screen for growth hormone deficiency. IGF-1 levels can, however, be low in malnutrition and in liver disease.

A 57. **A.** false **B.** false **C.** true **D.** false **E.** false

Varicella zoster virus vaccine is a live vaccine, and therefore is contraindicated in immunocompromised children and during pregnancy. A newborn infant whose mother developed chicken pox within 2 days prior to and 5 days post-delivery is at risk of developing severe disease and will not have received any protective maternal antibodies. They should be treated with varicella zoster immunoglobulin (VZIG) and, if vesicles develop, also with aciclovir.

A 58. **A.** false **B.** false **C.** true **D.** true **E.** true

Cat scratch disease is due to infection with *Bartonella henselae*. It is most commonly due to a scratch from a kitten, but infection may enter via the eye, thought to be from rubbing the eye after contact with a cat, causing a conjunctivitis and rarely a granulomatous lesion on the palpebral conjunctiva. The disease can become disseminated with fever, malaise, myalgia, arthralgia and abdominal pain. Granulomatous lesions may be found in the liver and spleen.

A **59.** **A.** false **B.** true **C.** true **D.** true **E.** false

Adenovirus, rubella, cytomegalovirus, *Toxoplasma gondii* and HHV-6 can all present with an infectious mononucleosis-type picture.

A **60.** **A.** true **B.** true **C.** true **D.** true **E.** true

Other infections that can cause an atypical lymphocytosis include viral hepatitis, malaria and mycoplasma.

'Best of five' questions

FOR EACH QUESTION, SELECT ONE ANSWER ONLY

Q 1. A 2-week-old baby of a mother with advanced HIV infection has proven CMV pneumonia. The drug of choice for treatment is

A. Aciclovir
B. Caspofungin
C. Voriconazole
D. Ganciclovir
E. Beta-interferon

Q 2. You are treating a 3-year-old girl from London with clinical signs and radiological evidence of a lower lobe pneumonia. The pathogen most likely to cause this picture in the UK is

A. *Moraxella catarrhalis*
B. Respiratory syncytial virus
C. *Streptococcus pneumoniae*
D. *Staphylococcus aureus*
E. *Mycobacterium tuberculosis*

Q 3. A child on immunosuppressive treatment post-liver transplant is known to be varicella zoster virus (VZV) antibody seronegative. She has been at nursery where several children have been diagnosed with what appears to be chicken pox. Which of the following is the best next course of action

A. Give intravenous immunoglobulin
B. Give a 7-day course of oral aciclovir
C. Admit for observation
D. Give VZIG
E. Give oral aciclovir and VZIG

Q 4. A 2-year-old boy recently returned from Pakistan is suspected of having *Giardia* infection. Which of the following statements best fits the clinical features of infection with *Giardia*

A. *Giardia* is commonly symptomatic
B. *Giardia* is an infection of the upper small intestine
C. *Giardia* rarely causes malabsorption of fats
D. *Giardia lamblia* commonly migrates to the bile ducts
E. *Giardia* infection is more prevalent in Europe compared to resource-poor countries.

Extended matching question

Options

A. Measles
B. Rheumatic fever
C. Scarlet fever
D. Staphylococcal scalded skin syndrome
E. Juvenile rheumatoid arthritis
F. Kawasaki disease
G. Leptospirosis
H. Adenovirus infection
I. Glandular fever
J. Hepatitis A
K. Falciparum malaria
L. Typhoid fever

For the patient described below, select the <u>single</u> most likely diagnosis from the list of options above. Each option may be used once, more than once or not at all.

Q 1.   A previously fit and well girl aged 5 years presents with a 1-week history of fever and extreme irritability. On examination she has conjunctivitis, a polymorphic rash and left knee swelling.

Bloods reveal the following:	Haemoglobin	12.0 g/dl
	White cell count	7.2
	Platelets	505×10^9/l
	CRP	70
	ESR	90
	Rheumatoid factor	negative
Urine culture:	Less than 50 white blood cells	
	No organisms isolated	

A1.   F. (Kawasaki disease)

'Best of five' questions

A 1. **D.**

A 2. **C.**

Streptococcus pneumoniae is the most common bacterial pathogen worldwide in children. It is the commonest cause of community-acquired pneumonia in the UK. They are predominantly sensitive to penicillin.

A 3. **E.**

The child, who is immunosuppressed and not immune to varicella zoster virus has been exposed to the virus. She should be given both oral aciclovir and varicella zoster immunoglobulin (VZIG).

A 4. **B.**

Giardia is a parasitic infection that may be symptomless. It is transferred via the faecal-oral route. Other symptoms include flatulence, diarrhoea, nausea/vomiting and greasy stools. Treatment is metronidazole or tinidazole with symptomatic management. It is estimated that up to 20% of the world's population is infected with *Giardia lamblia*.

Extended matching question

A 1. **F.** (Kawasaki disease)

'Best of five' questions

FOR EACH QUESTION, SELECT ONE ANSWER ONLY

Q 1. In a child with suspected Kawasaki disease (KD), which of the following is the best course of action

   A. Aspirin should be started based on the platelet count.
   B. intravenous immunoglobulin (IVIG) should ideally be started within 10 days.
   C. A second dose of IVIG should never be given
   D. Children with a normal ECHO in the first week should stop taking aspirin
   E. Aspirin treatment should never continue for more than a month

Q 2. Of the following, only one is true of Leptospirosis infection

   A. Infection is more common in children than adults
   B. Leptospira prefer cold climates
   C. The incubation period is 4–6 weeks
   D. It is related to rodents' urine in urban environments
   E. Person-to-person spread is common

Q 3. A 10-year-old boy recently returned from a camping trip has a red macular lesion which has expanded to become a large irregular annular lesion. He is febrile and has joint pain. Which organism is the most likely pathogen

   A. *Borrelia recurrentis*
   B. *Bordetella pertussis*
   C. *Borrelia burgdorferi*
   D. *Brucella melitensis*
   E. *Burkholderia pseudomallei*

Q 4. A 3-year-old boy who visited his family in Ghana presents with a fever of 1 week and 2 days of headache and sleepiness on his return to the UK. His Glasgow Coma Scale score is 10 out of 15. He looks unwell but there are no signs of meningitis. Your next course of action would be

    A. Arrange an urgent CT scan of the brain

    B. Check FBC, blood cultures, CRP and start intravenous cefotaxime

    C. After taking FBC, CRP and blood cultures perform a lumbar puncture to exclude meningitis

    D. Take FBC, blood cultures, CRP and malaria film and start intravenous quinine

    E. Take a FBC, CRP, malaria films and give oral chloroquine

Extended matching question

Options

  A. Measles
  B. Rheumatic fever
  C. Scarlet fever
  D. Staphylococcal scalded skin syndrome
  E. Juvenile rheumatoid arthritis
  F. Kawasaki disease
  G. Leptospirosis
  H. Adenovirus infection
  I. Glandular fever
  J. Hepatitis A
  K. Falciparum malaria
  L. Typhoid fever

For the patient described below, select the single most likely diagnosis from the list of options above. Each option may be used once, more than once or not at all.

Q 1. A 3-year-old girl who is previously healthy presents with a limp. There is no relevant family history. On examination she has a swollen and tender right knee. Her temperature is 37.8 °C. She has a polymorphic rash and cervical lymphadenopathy.

Bloods reveal the following:

Haemoglobin •	14.0 g/dl
White cell count	9.0
Platelets	$586 \times 10^9/l$
Neutrophils	2.8
CRP	15
ESR	98
Rheumatoid factor	Negative
Urea and electrolytes	normal

Knee aspirate: Negative for pus cells and organisms.

A1.   **E.** (Juvenile idiopathic arthritis)

'Best of five' questions

A 1.   B.

Once a diagnosis of KD has been made it is vital that IVIG is given asap but ideally before 10 days to reduce the risk of coronary artery aneurysms (CAAs). However it is still recommended that IVIG is given at diagnosis, even if after 10 days. In untreated KD 20–40% of KD will develop CAAs. Half of these will regress within 5 years.

A 2.   D.

Leptospira cause a systemic illness that often leads to renal and hepatic dysfunction. The organism enters the body when mucous membranes or abraded skin comes in contact with contaminated environmental sources. The most important reservoirs are rodents, and rats are the most common source worldwide. The incubation period is usually 7–12 days, with a range of 2–20 days. Approximately 90% of patients manifest a mild anicteric form of the disease, and approximately 5–10% have the severe form with jaundice, otherwise known as Weil disease. The natural course of leptospirosis falls into two distinct phases, septicaemic and immune. During a brief period of 1–3 days between the two phases, the patient shows some improvement.

A 3.   C.

Lyme disease is due to infection with the spirochete, *Borrelia burgdorferi*, and the body's immune response to it. It is transmitted by the bite of *Ixodes* ticks. Erythema chronicum migrans is an annular erythematous lesion that increases in size over several days, which can be asymptomatic, itchy or burn, occuring at or near the site of the tick bite such as the axilla or groin. The infection can than go on to give an inflammatory arthritis with cranial nerve palsies, carditis, malaise and fatigue.

A 4.   **D.**

This child is at risk of malaria and is showing signs of cerebral malaria. Whilst all the other options may be considered he requires confirmation of malaria with thick and thin films and starting IV quinine. He will require close neurological observations and monitoring blood glucose levels, with repeat blood films and a parasitaemia count until the clear.

Extended matching question

A 1.   **E.** (Juvenile idiopathic arthritis)

'Best of five' questions

FOR EACH QUESTION, SELECT <u>ONE</u> ANSWER ONLY

Q 1. Which of the following statements is most accurate concerning mumps infection in children?

   A. Mumps infection is a rare cause of deafness caused by infections in the UK
   B. Orchitis is the most common symptom in boys
   C. Mumps is common in infants less than 1 year of age
   D. Bilateral parotitis is the most common symptom in children
   E. Mumps nephritis is a leading cause of renal problems in children.

Q 2. Regarding non-tuberculosis (atypical) mycobacterial disease in children, which of the following is most accurate

   A. It is always transmitted from person to person
   B. Contact tracing is vital in suspected cases
   C. NTM lymphadenitis is most common in pre-school children
   D. The incubation period is 3–4 days
   E. It should be treated with rifampicin, isoniazid and oral pyrazinamide

Q 3. Fifth disease (slapped cheek syndrome) is caused by Parvovirus B19; which of the following is most accurate

   A. It is a small, non-enveloped DNA virus
   B. It is more common in adults
   C. It is asymptomatic in 90% of cases
   D. It commonly causes an aplastic crisis
   E. Aciclovir can be an effective treatment

Q 4. Which organism is the most likely pathogen in a 10-week-old boy with a worsening dry, paroxysmal cough, vomiting and recurrent apnoeas?

A. Metapneumovirus
B. Respiratory syncytial virus
C. *Bordetella pertussis*
D. *Mycoplasma pneumoniae*
E. Adenovirus

Extended matching question

Options

A. Measles
B. Rheumatic fever
C. Scarlet fever
D. Staphylococcal scalded skin syndrome
E. Juvenile rheumatoid arthritis
F. Kawasaki disease
G. Leptospirosis
H. Adenovirus infection
I. Glandular fever
J. Hepatitis A
K. Falciparum malaria
L. Typhoid fever

For the patient described below, select the <u>single</u> most likely diagnosis from the list of options above. Each option may be used once, more than once or not at all.

Q 1. **An 8-year-old boy originally from Pakistan presents with a 10-day history of watery diarrhoea, and for the last 3 days vomiting. On examination he is miserable, mildly dehydrated and has a non-specific maculopapular rash on his trunk and arms.**

Bloods reveal the following:	Haemoglobin1	2.5 gm/dl
	White cell count	12.0
	Platelets	$340 \times 10^9/l$
	Neutrophils	3.4
	Lymphocytes	7.1
	Sodium	146
	Potassium	3.0
	Urea	7.5
	Creatinine	57
Stool culture:	Negative for bacteria and parasites
Urine microscopy:	Normal
A1.	H. (Adenovirus infection)

'Best of five' questions

A 1. **D.**

The mumps virus is a paramyxovirus. Humans are the sole reservoir for the mumps virus, and the transmission mode is via respiratory droplets from person to person. Unilateral hearing loss is associated with mumps infection but is rare. Approximately 10% of all infected patients develop a mild form of meningitis; encephalitis, transient myelitis, or polyneuritis is rare. Orchitis occurs in 10–20% of patients. Subsequent sterility is rare. Other uncommon complications include myocarditis, nephritis, arthritis, thyroiditis, pancreatitis, thrombocytopenia purpura, mastitis, and pneumonia. These usually resolve within 2–3 weeks without sequelae.

A 2. **C.**

A 3. **A.**

Parvovirus B19, a member of the family *Parvoviridae*, is a heat-stable, single-stranded DNA virus. The incubation period is usually 7–10 days but can be 4–21 days. Fifth disease or Erythema infectiosum is usually a biphasic illness. Mild prodromal symptoms begin approximately 1 week after exposure and last 2–3 days. These symptoms precede a symptom-free period of about 7–10 days, followed by a typical exanthem that occurs in three stages:

1. A bright red, raised, slapped-cheek rash with circumoral pallor develops, sparing the nasolabial folds.
2. This phase occurs 1–4 days later and is characterized by an erythematous maculopapular rash on proximal extremities (usually arms and extensor surfaces) and trunk, which fades into a classic lace-like reticular pattern as confluent areas clear. The palms and soles usually are spared.

3. Frequent recurrences can occur for weeks and may be due to stimuli such as exercise, irritation, or overheating of skin from bathing or sunlight.

Treatment is supportive.

[A] **4.** **C.**

Humans are the sole reservoir for *B. pertussis* and *B. parapertussis*. The incubation period for the organism is typically 7–10 days. Pertussis has 3 stages, each lasting from 1 to 2 weeks. Stage 1 is the initial (catarrhal) phase and is indistinguishable from common upper respiratory infections with low-grade fever. Stage 2 presents with paroxysms of intense coughing lasting up to several minutes. In older infants and toddlers, the paroxysms of coughing sometimes are followed by a loud whoop as inspired air passes through a still partially closed airway. Infants less than 6 months do not have the characteristic whoop but may present with apnoeic episodes. Post-cough vomiting and turning red with coughing are common in affected children. Stage 3 may involve a chronic cough, lasting up to several weeks.

Extended matching question

[A] **1.** **H.** (Adenovirus infection)

'Best of five' questions

FOR EACH QUESTION, SELECT <u>ONE</u> ANSWER ONLY

Q 1. Which one of the following commonly causes an aplastic crisis in a child suffering from sickle cell disease?

  A. Herpes simplex virus
  B. Influenza A virus
  C. Respiratory syncytial virus
  D. Parvovirus
  E. Metapneumovirus

Q 2. In vertically acquired HIV infection in children, which is the most common opportunistic infection

  A. *Cryptococcus meningitis*
  B. CMV infection
  C. *Pneumocystis carinii* pneumonia
  D. *Escherichia coli* urinary tract infection
  E. *Mycobacterium tuberculosis*

Q 3. A mother who is 40 weeks pregnant develops clinical signs of chicken pox (varicella zoster infection) 2 days before her healthy baby is born. Which of the following is the best course of action

  A. Advise the mother to stop breast-feeding and give her oral aciclovir
  B. The baby should be given oral aciclovir and discharged with no follow-up
  C. The baby should be nursed on an open ward and given oral aciclovir
  D. The baby should receive varicella zoster immunoglobulin (VZIG) intramuscularly and followed-up

E. VZV antibody status should be checked in the baby and follow-up arranged

Q 4. **Which of the following statements best describes the mode of transmission of *Mycobacterium tuberculosis* infection?**

A. Communicability is highest from untreated pulmonary infection
B. Young children with tuberculosis are commonly infectious.
C. The tubercle bacillus is usually passed on via stool or urine in cases of household transmission
D. Transmission is commonly via salivary secretions
E. Prolonged close contact (household) rarely causes tuberculosis (TB) infection in children

Extended matching question

Options

A. Measles
B. Rheumatic fever
C. Scarlet fever
D. Staphylococcal scalded skin syndrome
E. Juvenile rheumatoid arthritis
F. Kawasaki disease
G. Leptospirosis
H. Adenovirus infection
I. Glandular fever
J. Hepatitis A
K. Falciparum malaria
L. Typhoid fever

For the patient described below, select the single most likely diagnosis from the list of options above. Each option may be used once, more than once or not at all.

Q 1. **A 14-year-old girl has recently returned from an activity week at a watersports centre in the Lake District. She complains of a 5-day history of fever, rigors and a maculopapular rash on her trunk, back and limbs. Several days later she develops a yellow discolouration of her skin. On examination she is irritable and lethargic with a temperature of 37.9 °C. She has small, non-tender cervical lymph nodes.**

Bloods reveal the following:

Haemoglobin	10.8 g/dl
White cell count	13.0
Platelets	$400 \times 10^9/l$
Neutrophils	5.5
Lymphocytes	4.0
Eosinophils	0.7
Sodium	138
Potassium	3.4
Urea	4.4
Creatinine	50
CRP	67
ESR	50
ALT	92
ALP	700
Bilirubin	57
Albumin	32

Urine culture:	NAD
Blood culture:	NAD
Stool culture:	NAD
A1.	**G.** (Leptospirosis)

'Best of five' questions

A 1.   **D.**

Parvovirus B19, the only member of the *Parvoviridae* family known to cause disease in humans, is a single-strand DNA virus. It commonly causes Erythema infectiosum in children, a mild viral illness followed by a classic exanthem in which both cheeks appear bright red as though they had been slapped, hence the name slapped cheek syndrome. In patients with haemoglobinopathies or haemolytic anemias, because the duration of erythrocyte survival is decreased, a decrease in the reticulocyte count to less than 1% can lead to an aplastic crisis. It is characterized by a profound anaemia caused by a temporary halt in new erythrocyte production. B19V is the only known infectious cause of aplastic crisis.

A 2.   **C.**

Any of the others can occur but PCP is commonest. MTB infections are more common in the extremely rare gamma-interferon deficiency.

A 3.   **D.**

It is debatable whether oral aciclovir should be given as well as the VZIG. The aim is to reduce the risk of severe disseminated varicella infection. Some centres recommend both. The child certainly needs follow-up to monitor the complications. Maternal chicken pox infection in early to mid-pregnancy is estimated to have a 1–2% risk of causing the congenital varicella syndrome, which is characterized by limb hypoplasia, muscular atrophy, skin scarring, cortical atrophy, microcephaly, cataract formation and rudimentary digits.

A 4.   **A.**

Tuberculosis (TB) is the most common cause of infection-related death worldwide. In 1993, the World Health Organization (WHO) declared TB to be a global public health emergency. *Mycobacterium tuberculosis* is the most common cause of TB. The acid-fast characteristic of the mycobacteria is their unique feature. TB occurs when individuals inhale bacteria aerosolized by infected persons. The organism is slow growing and tolerates the intracellular environment, where it may remain inert for years before reactivation and disease. The main determinant of the pathogenicity of TB is its ability to escape host defence mechanisms, including macrophages and delayed hypersensitivity responses. Immunosuppression increases risk of developing disease. Pulmonary TB may manifest itself in several forms, including endobronchial TB with focal lymphadenopathy, progressive pulmonary disease, pleural involvement, and reactivated pulmonary disease. Symptoms of primary pulmonary disease in the paediatric population can be subtle or non-existent. Symptoms are more likely to occur in infants such as fever, night sweats, anorexia, non-productive cough and failure to thrive, and difficulty gaining weight may occur. Extrapulmonary TB includes peripheral lymphadenopathy, tubercular meningitis, miliary TB, skeletal TB and other organ involvement. Key to diagnosis is obtaining appropriate specimens for bacteriologic examination. Examination of sputum, gastric lavage, bronchoalveolar lavage, lung tissue, lymph node tissue, bone marrow, blood, liver, CSF, urine and stool may be useful, depending on the location of the disease. Gastric aspirates are used in lieu of sputum in very young children (<6 years) who usually do not have a cough deep enough to produce sputum for analysis. Conventional methods include the Ziehl-Neelsen staining method. PCR can be used. Chest radiograph is the diagnostic tool when evaluating patients for pulmonary TB with microbiological confirmation of bronchial washings during bronchoscopy. Screening uses the internationally recognized Mantoux test, using tuberculin PPD given intradermally. Treatment of MTB involves first-line agents such as rifampin, isoniazid (INH), pyrazinamide, ethambutol, and streptomycin. Follow local protocols but it usually involves three or four drugs for 3 months followed by two agents for a further 3–4 months. Courses of treatment must be completed to reduce the risk of antibiotic resistance. Current treatment is being complicated by multi-drug resistant MTB.

Extended matching question

[A] 1.   **G.** (Leptospirosis)

'Best of five' questions

FOR EACH QUESTION, SELECT <u>ONE</u> ANSWER ONLY

Q 1. Which of the following statements is most accurate concerning hepatitis C infection in children?

    A. Coexisting HIV infection in the mother does not increase the risk of hepatitis C transmission to the newborn

    B. Most current hepatitis C infections in the UK are caused by contaminated blood products

    C. Risk of needle-stick transmission is about 90%

    D. Transmission through sexual intercourse is common

    E. Most patients will develop liver cirrhosis within 10 years

Q 2. In *Neisseria meningitidis* infection which one of the following is most accurate

    A. The incubation period is 2–10 days

    B. It rarely causes meningitis

    C. Nasopharyngeal carriage is eradicated by all antibiotics

    D. It is not a notifiable disease in the UK

    E. it is carried in the nasopharynx of domestic animals

Q 3. A 1-week-old baby presents with poor feeding and is pyrexial at 38.0 °C. On examination she is pale, irritable and has a runny nose. She is tachycardic at 190 bpm and has a central capillary refill time of 4 seconds. She has a maculopapular rash with crusted lesions on her palms and soles of her feet and significant hepatosplenomegaly. Which is the most likely pathogen

    A. Herpes simplex virus

    B. *Treponema pallidum*

    C. Group B streptococcus
    D. *Escherichia coli*
    E. *Listeria monocytogenes*

Q 4. ***Leishmania donovani* causes visceral leishmaniasis in children from tropical and sub-tropical regions. Which of the following is the insect vector for the disease**

    A. *Culex mosquito*
    B. *Ixode* tick
    C. *Ascaris lumbricoides*
    D. Sandfly
    E. Simulian blackfly

Extended matching question

Options

A. Measles
B. Rheumatic fever
C. Scarlet fever
D. Staphylococcal scalded skin syndrome
E. Juvenile rheumatoid arthritis
F. Kawasaki disease
G. Leptospirosis
H. Adenovirus infection
I. Glandular fever
J. Hepatitis A
K. Falciparum malaria
L. Typhoid fever

For the patient described below, select the <u>single</u> most likely diagnosis from the list of options above. Each option may be used once, more than once or not at all.

Q 1. **A 7-year-old girl has returned from a family trip to Goa, India 3 weeks ago. She complains of an intermittent fever, feeling unwell and has not passed any stool for four days. On examination she is febrile and lethargic, has a 3 cm spleen palpable. Her pulse is regular, blood pressure 90/53 mmHg and heart rate 50 bpm.**

Bloods reveal the following:

Haemoglobin	10.5 g/dl
White cell count	15.2
Platelets	$288 \times 10^9/l$
Urea & electrolytes:	Normal
LFTs:	Normal
CRP:	44
ESR:	20

Urine:	NAD
Malaria screen:	Negative
A1.	**M.** (Typhoid fever)

Exam 5 — Supplementary Answers

'Best of five' questions

A 1. **B.**

The risk of needle-stick injury is about 3%.

A 2. **A.**

Invasion of the bloodstream by *Neisseria meningitidis* causes a spectrum of diseases ranging from a fatal overwhelming infection to a transient bacteraemia that is relatively benign. The human nasopharynx is the only known reservoir of meningococcal infection. Meningococci spread from person to person by airborne droplets of infected nasopharyngeal secretions. The clinical pattern of meningococcaemia is varied. A skin rash, which is essential for recognizing meningococcaemia, may advance from a few ill-defined lesions to a widespread petechial eruption within a few hours. Fulminant meningococcaemia is the most serious form of meningococcal disease. It begins abruptly with a high fever, myalgias/weakness, nausea, vomiting and headache. The rash appears suddenly and is widespread, purpuric and ecchymotic. The underlying pathology is capillary leak syndrome with activation of the inflammatory and clotting cascade leading to DIC and intravascular fluid depletion. The mainstay of treatment is aggressive fluid resuscitation and antibiotics and transfer to an intensive care unit.

A 3. **B.**

Congenital syphilis is caused by transplacental or peripartum transmission of spirochaetes. Perinatal death may result from congenital infection in more than 40% of affected, untreated pregnancies. Traditionally congenital infection has been divided into early (within the first 2 years) and late (after 2 years) stages. The typical stillborn or highly symptomatic newborn is born prematurely with hepatosplenomegaly, skeletal involvement, and often pneumonia and bullous skin lesions. The earliest signs of congenital syphilis may be poor feeding and snuffles (syphilitic rhinitis). Complications include neurosyphilis and involvement of the teeth, bones, eyes and the VIIIth cranial nerve. Follow-up for development and hearing/vision is vital.

A 4.   D.

Culex mosquito transmits malaria, the *Ixodes* tick transmits *Borrelia burgdorferi* (Lyme disease), *Ascaris* a helminth intestinal infection, Simulian blackfly transmits oncocerciasis (river blindness).

Extended matching question

A 1.   M. (Typhoid fever)